Of Acceptable Risk

SCIENCE AND THE DETERMINATION OF SAFETY

William W. Lowrance

HARVARD UNIVERSITY

William Kaufmann, Inc.   Los Altos, California

To those who wrestle honestly with these issues

and

To those who have encouraged, taught, and tolerated,
especially among them my mother and father

Library of Congress Cataloging in Publication Data

Lowrance, William W   1943-
    Of acceptable risk.

    Includes bibliographical references.
    1. Product safety. 2. Industrial safety.
I. Title.
TS175.L68   363   76-834
ISBN 0-913232-30-0
ISBN 0-913232-31-9 pbk.

Copyright © 1976 by William Kaufmann, Inc.

Printed in the United States of America

Contents

Foreword

The safety of the public has become a critical issue of public debate and has been the subject of extensive reporting in the daily press and other media. It has been our observation that some of this reporting is not sufficiently informed, especially as concerns the scientific basis—and limitations—of the determination of safety and of the role of scientists in this process.

The Committee on Science and Public Policy of the National Academy of Sciences had become concerned over these issues; it was fortunate to discover that Dr. William W. Lowrance, who was coming to the Academy as an Alfred P. Sloan Foundation Resident Fellow, was also interested in the problem and was willing to dedicate his full attention to the writing of this book. We hope that the analysis and interpretation presented in the following pages will be interesting and useful to those involved in the legislative process and in the popularization of the complex issues involved in the determination of safety.

This book was written by Bill Lowrance; however, throughout its preparation he consulted the *ad hoc* panel listed below, appointed by the Committee on Science and Public Policy, on matters of organization, conceptual content, balance, format, and expression. We enjoyed that exchange, which was both lively and productive. Although we do not necessarily endorse every view expressed here, we believe that the ideas are thoughtfully and engagingly presented and are worthy of serious consideration. We commend their careful study to everyone concerned about these important problems.

H. S. GUTOWSKY, *chairman of the Panel on Science and the Determination of Safety,*
Committee on Science and Public Policy,
National Academy of Sciences
and
Professor of Chemistry, University of Illinois

PANEL MEMBERS:

RAYMOND BOWERS
Professor of Physics
Director of the Program on Science, Technology and Society
Cornell University

HARVEY BROOKS
Benjamin Peirce Professor of Technology and Public Policy
Harvard University

PETER GOLDMAN
Professor of Clinical Pharmacology
Harvard Medical School

G. B. KISTIAKOWSKY
Emeritus Professor of Chemistry
Harvard University

HERSCHEL L. ROMAN
Professor of Genetics
University of Washington

Author's Preface

It was my very good fortune when I arrived at the National Academy of Sciences in mid-1973 as a Sloan Foundation Resident Fellow to find that a number of my interests were shared by members of the Committee on Science and Public Policy. Prominent among our mutual interests was a concern for the notion of safety, which is central to a great many issues but has so far been poorly defined, widely misunderstood, and often misrepresented. We decided to study the issues intensively and prepare the present book. The inspiration for the project was G. B. Kistiakowsky's, who from the very beginning imparted guidance to the endeavor with the remarkable energies and critical skills for which he has always been known. The agreement was that I would work as an independent scholar, pursuing the issues wherever they led me and writing whatever had to be written, trying out ideas on an informal panel appointed by the Committee on Science and Public Policy. The panel commented on my drafts, opened doors, and in general tried to keep me out of trouble. All along, the Committee on Science and Public Policy hosted my work and provided thoughtful guidance. From my point of view the arrangement could not have been more cordial or effective. I am grateful to the Alfred P. Sloan Foundation for providing my fellowship, and to the National Science Foundation for underwriting the project.

The members of the panel have asked me not to toss them bouquets; no matter: the quality of their contributions will readily be appreciated by everyone who knows these men. I will always be grateful for their encouragement and trust—and for their not charging tuition.

It is an author's privilege to register his debts in his preface; I do so now, sincerely and with much pleasure: to the many people who, through patient discussion and blue-penciling, helped shape these ideas; to Robert E. Green, Judy Marshall, Amahl Shakhashiri, and John R. Underwood, my colleagues of the staff of the Committee on Science and Public Policy; to Celine Alvey, Peggy McArtor, James Olson, and Marilyn Urion, of the Academy library, relentless trackers of information; and, for personal reasons known to them, to David Z. Beckler, Paul Doty, Robert Hume, Robert N. Kreidler, David L. Luck, Jan Amy Rostov, and Greta Schuessler.

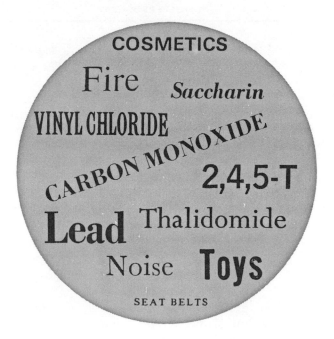

1
The Safety Problem

Few headlines are so alarming, perplexing, and personal in their implications as those concerning safety. Frightening stories jolt our early morning complacency so frequently that we wonder whether things can really be *that* bad. We are disturbed by what sometimes appear to be haphazard and irresponsible regulatory actions, and we can't help being suspicious of all the assaults on our freedoms and our pocketbooks made in the name of safety. We hardly know which cries of "Wolf!" to respond to; but we dare not forget that even in the fairy tale, the wolf really did come.

The issues: X-rays, cosmetics, DDT, lead, pharmaceuticals, toys, saccharin, intrauterine contraceptive devices, power lawn mowers, air pollutants, noise. . . .

1

The questions: How do we determine how hazardous these things are? Why is it that cyclamates one day dominate the market as the principal calorie-cutting sweetener in millions of cans of diet drinks, only to be banned the next day because there is a "very slight chance" they may cause cancer? Why is it that one group of eminent experts says that medical X-rays (or food preservatives, or contraceptive pills) are safe and ought to be used more widely, while another group of authorities, equally reputable, urges that exposure to the same things should be restricted because they are unsafe? At what point do debates such as that over DDT stop being scientific and objective and start being political and subjective? How can anyone gauge the public's willingness to accept risks? Why must there be these endless controversies over such things as lead, whose effects on health have been known in detail for years? Are people being irresponsible, or is there something about these problems that just naturally spawns confusion? Just what sort of a decisionmaking tool is this notion of "safety"?

Exploring these problems, and the underlying concept of safety itself, is the purpose of this book. We believe that if certain pervasive themes are properly appreciated, the whole field of safety will be better understood. This presentation is an attempt to stimulate thought and debate on those themes. Rather than trying to resolve any particular product- or environmental–safety questions, it deals with question-asking itself. Its principal emphasis is on the contributions of scientists and other technically trained people, but it also describes the general features of the social context within which safety decisions are made. It does not attempt to evaluate the work of particular institutions, agencies, or individuals.

Principles are illustrated with real examples selected for their explanatory usefulness. The problems used for illustration are all of intense current public interest; many of them, such as radiation, DDT, pharmaceuticals, and noise, have a long history as well. Few of them are novel or "exotic"; indeed, some, such as baby cribs, bicycles, and cosmetics, are included deliberately because they seem so prosaic. We could have chosen any of hundreds of other examples. Some very important public problems such as nuclear reactors and automobile traffic safety have been given only passing reference because they are so complex, both technically and politically, that they would not illustrate the fundamental principles as clearly as the examples we have used.

Our examples are "for instances" given in enough detail to illustrate specific points. In using an action as an illustration, we are not necessarily approving of it; we are simply describing what has happened, using the case to exemplify question-asking and problem-solving. For those who wish to pursue particular issues further, we have provided references to readily available source materials.

Writings on safety tend to leave a gloomy impression that everything is dismayingly unsafe. Every age has its hazards; ours has devised some alarming new ones—such as artificially generated radiation—in addition to those, such as water pollution, that have plagued man through the ages. But it must be remembered that we have conquered many of the classical threats to human health and are continually acquiring better understanding of those that still elude our control.

This study takes the following as points of departure: (1) technology, although by no means an unmixed blessing, has in many ways enriched the human condition and will long remain an important aspect of civilization; (2) many of our problems are technological in origin and will necessarily be technological, as well as political, in their solution; (3) human activity will always and unavoidably involve risks; and (4) in order to make our world safer, we can start changing only from where things are today.

It must be kept in mind that not all hazards are manmade. Technology does not always deserve the blame. Man has forever had to contend not only with natural catastrophes and infectious diseases, but also with nutritional deficiencies, natural water and air pollution, allergies to such agents as poison ivy and ragweed pollen, poisoning from chemicals in mushrooms and in many other natural foods, and the ravages of sun, wind, sand, earthquake, drought, flood, fire, and frost. Technological development has indeed brought undesirable effects, but many of these must be viewed as the expense of decreasing our vulnerability to the hazards of nature.

THE HAZARDS CHANGE

Mankind is in many ways safer today than ever before. At least, the hazards change. To make comparison, no need to go back to the cavemen, who, the jawbone record tells us, spent their days in unrelieved pain from chronic toothache. No need to look at the Middle Ages, whose pestilences settled on hundreds of thousands of people at a time. No need, either, to go back to the grim factory towns of the industrial revolution, where dangerously exposed machinery and smoke-clogged alleys consumed men just as surely as the cotton fields and coal mines did. But for perspective, think for just a moment about the opening years of the present century.

In 1900 the principal insecticide, sprayed on everything from apples and grapes to strawberries and potatoes, was "Paris green"—lead

3

arsenate.[1] The first canned foods were being preserved with sulfites, boric acid, and formaldehyde at rather high concentrations. The leading anti-septic for home and hospital use was corrosive carbolic acid. The red robustness of teas, candies, and other commercial food products was imparted by lead chromate, which today's biochemist would prefer not even to handle, much less feed to anybody. Medicinals were unreliable: "Adulteration threatened the healing art. Even more alarming was the spread of proprietary or patent medicines. Some had genuine merit, but most were nostrums, often containing dangerous, habit-forming ingredients. Such fraudulent remedies were far from new, but in the latter part of the 19th century they increased in number and resort to consumption cures, lost-manhood tonics, soothing syrups, liver pills, and other so-called remedies became a craze."[2] Foods were often adulterated; the laws controlling food composition were weak. Tinctures of opium such as laudanum and paregoric were readily available in corner drugstores and were unchecked from indiscriminate use. Children frequently became habituated.

As to the general environment, some rivers were so filthy with raw sewage and industrial waste that, as the saying went, "bait died on the hook." Industrial towns were black with coal soot, as were people's lungs. Workers labored at their own peril.

In a "modest personal attempt to redeem our times from the aspersions cast upon them by nostalgic comparisons," Otto L. Bettmann, founder of the Bettmann Archive in New York, has recently published, with commentary, some of the most poignant items from his pictorial archives. In this he vividly reminds us of some aspects of turn-of-the-century America that our selective cultural memory has preferred to forget: a New York with 150,000 horses in its streets; "kitchen slops, cinders, coal dust, horse manure, broken cobblestones and dumped merchandise" piled high on its sidewalks; a roaring, cinder-spitting "El" overhead; recurrent waves of diphtheria sweeping from the slums down the more fashionable avenues; and sweatshop exploitation of workers for whom there was no recourse.[3]

Urbanization, a burgeoning mass media, and an advertising industry that felt little obligation to truthfulness were opening a vast consumer market in such a way that in 1933 the reformer Arthur Kallet would

[1] James Clifton Whorton, Before Silent Spring (Princeton University Press, Princeton, N.J., 1974).

[2] Oscar E. Anderson, Jr., "Pioneer statute: The Pure Food and Drugs Act of 1906," Journal of Public Law 13, 189-196 (1964).

[3] Otto L. Bettmann, The Good Old Days — They Were Terrible! (Random House, N. Y., 1974).

look back on what had been happening and call the American people *100,000,000 Guinea Pigs*:

> In the magazines, in the newspapers, over the radio, a terrific verbal barrage has been laid down on a hundred million Americans, first, to set in motion a host of fears about their health, their stomachs, their bowels, their teeth, their throats, their looks; second, to persuade them that only by eating, drinking, gargling, brushing, or smearing with Smith's Whole Vitamin Breakfast Food, Jones' Yeast Cubes, Blue Giant Apples, Prussian Salts, Listroboris Mouthwash, Grandpa's Wonder Toothpaste, and a thousand and one other foods, drinks, gargles, and pastes, can they either postpone the onset of disease, of social ostracism, of business failure, or recover from ailments, physical or social, already contracted.[4]

Farm families were not immune to all this, since, being far from doctors and depending on mail-ordered restoratives, liniments, balms, and other patent curatives, they were prime targets for promotional assaults. For rural America, which in 1900 was the majority of the population, unceasing vigilance was necessary in contending with the hazards of axes, mules, stinging insects, boiling laundry kettles, tetanus-inducing rusty implements and barbed wire, impure water, and spoiled food.

The principal fatal diseases were pneumonia, influenza, and tuberculosis. Infant mortality was high; in 1900, more than thirteen percent of all American children died before their first birthday.

No need to belabor the point; in many ways we are better off than we used to be. In a sense we now have the luxury to worry about subtle hazards which at one time, even if detected, would have been given only low priority beside the much greater hazards of the day. Whereas once the outright poison, lead arsenate, was at issue, we have come through several generations of much less toxic agents and now worry about what may be marginal effects of our current pesticides. We have largely gotten lead out of our food; the worst we have to contend with now is an occasional trace dissolving into food from a lead-soldered can seam. But the canning art itself has improved so much that cases of food poisoning, once common, are now so rare as to make the front pages of newspapers. As we worry about the disinfectant hexachlorophene in soap, we should also remember the harsh carbolic acid it has replaced and the surgical operations it has made safer; and, incidentally, we should be grateful for the retirement of that backyard hazard, the lye pot. Surely no case needs to be made for the public health and pharmaceutical revolutions—the conquering

---

[4]Arthur Kallet and F. J. Schlink, *100,000,000 Guinea Pigs*, 3 (Vanguard, New York, 1933).

in this country of malaria and typhoid and smallpox and polio and tuberculosis and the nutritional deficiency diseases. By comparison with the rickets and pellagra of ages not long past, our anxieties over supplemental vitamins and weight-reducing artificial sweeteners seem trivial. There are signs that our great rivers, lakes, and urban atmospheres are clearing, even if distressingly slowly. The move toward making our workplaces less hazardous is gaining momentum. Consumers have found collective strength, and *caveat emptor* no longer strictly governs the market. In the United States infant mortality in the first year of life is now down from thirteen percent in 1900 to about two percent—a fivefold decrease in seventy-five years.

We don't mean to be overly sanguine; most certainly there are problems, many of them urgently demanding resolution. That is why we have written this book. But in the safety issue, historical perspective is particularly enlightening, leaving us viewing our contemporary condition, as the biologist René Dubos expresses it, as "despairing optimists."

Notice the many different, but interdependent, reasons for the progress sketched above. In part, scientific advance was responsible, bringing forward empirical evidence about the subtle risks of Paris green, lead chromate, and the early food preservatives. Technology provided less harsh antiseptics, devised more efficacious and less risky pesticides and pharmaceuticals, and—together with extraordinary medical and public health innovations—established a rational basis for health protection.

At the same time and partly because of scientific advance, people's values and expectations changed. Discomforting discoveries were forced by the extraordinary growth in our social and physical scale. We have been startled into profound realizations, no less profound for having become commonplace: that the balance of nature is much more precarious than we had presumed; that nature's complex web is easily rent by our clumsy passage; that "there is no longer any 'away' into which to throw things"; that it is crucial that we stop fouling our earthly nest; and that what we do today will affect not only ourselves, and not only our children, but our descendants for many generations to come.

Much of the change has been closely coupled to the mechanisms of government. The 1906 Pure Food and Drugs Act was passed to combat the atrocities of food and drug adulteration and fraud; subsequent replacements and amendments have greatly extended government regulation of the safety of food and food additives, pharmaceuticals, cosmetics, radiation, and medical devices. The 1947 Federal Insecticide, Fungicide, and Rodenticide Act brought those agricultural and public health chemicals under government scrutiny. So also with the Coal Mine Health and Safety Act (1969), the Clean Air Amendments (1970), the Occupational Health and Safety Act (1970), the Consumer Product Safety Act (1970), and many others. A bureaucracy, for which even the usual journalistic "vast" is inadequate, has grown to include a Food and Drug Administration, an Environmental Protection Agency, an Occupational Safety and Health Administration, a Consumer Product Safety Commission, and an assortment of other agencies charged with regulating the products we buy and the surroundings in which we live and work. Legislative and administrative developments have evolved apace with social values as reflected in court determinations of the rights of workers, the liabilities of manufacturers, and the assignment of responsibilities for preserving the environment. Most evaluations of the efficacy and efficiency of these changes are mixed. To be sure, some of these developments have succeeded in protecting individuals from threats against which they would otherwise be defenseless. But others have simply compounded the problems, strewn red tape, and advanced the bureaucratization of society.

We would be remiss not to add the following note. Although we have indeed conquered many of the classical scourges and are in many ways better off than ever before, we currently find ourselves confronted by some new hazards that can fairly be said to appear "monstrous." They are problems which we don't yet know very much about: the radiation, steam explosion, theft, sabotage, and waste disposal hazards of the rapidly growing civilian nuclear power program; the poorly understood effects of attempts to modify the world's weather; the effects of freons and other manmade agents on the protective sunlight-filtering ozone shield of the upper atmosphere. Other such problems are being recognized. Their apparent monstrousness lies principally in their physical and temporal scale. The potential consequences are unprecedentedly widespread and terrible, indifferent to political boundaries. Some of these consequences may prove to be reversible only with great difficulty, with decades or even centuries having to pass before the mishap can be undone. We are now adopting many innovations for widespread use faster than we can even hope to learn about their consequences, thus tragically outsmarting ourselves. Further, the "scale of decisionmaking" involved here transcends that of all previous decisional situations except the uniquely bizarre ones of modern warfare; the decision of one small group can influence the well-being of an entire nation for many years to come, and what one nation decides can affect the fate of millions, or even billions, of unconsulted people around the world.

7

ORGANIZATION OF THIS BOOK

The remainder of the present chapter sketches the general nature of safety decisions, defining safety as a measure of the acceptability of risk. Chapter 2 presents the diverse problems of *Measuring Risk*. Then Chapter 3, *Judging Safety,* describes how the acceptability of risks is appraised. Chapter 4, *Safety Issues as Public Problems,* discusses personal roles, the functions of institutions, the development and resolution of controversies, and the issue of responsibility. *Making Safe,* Chapter 5, describes how knowledge and judgment are applied in devising safeguards. Chapter 6, *DDT: An Archetypal Modern Problem,* presents an extended example in which the issues raised in earlier chapters can be reviewed together. Then Chapter 7, *An Afterword,* brings the presentation to a close.

THE NATURE OF SAFETY DECISIONS

Much of the widespread confusion about the nature of safety decisions would be dispelled if the meaning of the term *safety* were clarified. For a concept so deeply rooted in both technical and popular usage, safety has remained dismayingly ill-defined.

We will define safety as a judgment of the acceptability of risk, and risk, in turn, as a measure of the probability and severity of harm to human health.

A thing is safe if its risks are judged to be acceptable.

By its preciseness and connotative power this definition contrasts sharply with simplistic dictionary definitions that have "safe" meaning something like "free from risk." Nothing can be absolutely free of risk. One can't think of anything that isn't, under some circumstances, able to cause harm. Because nothing can be absolutely free of risk, nothing can be said to be absolutely safe. There are degrees of risk, and consequently there are degrees of safety.

Notice that this definition emphasizes the relativity and judgmental nature of the concept of safety. It also implies that two very different activities are required for determining how safe things are: *measuring risk*, an objective but probabilistic pursuit; and *judging the acceptability of that risk (judging safety),* a matter of personal and social value judgment.

In scope, of course, these decisions range from the intensely personal to the broadly social, and, not necessarily respectively, from the whimsical and uninformed to the carefully analyzed and highly deliberate. The options available to individuals may in some cases be narrowed by considerations of physical scale, as with restraints on contamination of the environment, or of social scale, as with the standardization of consumer products available from giant manufacturing corporations.

The present text reflects the above definition of safety throughout, and develops the key terms "acceptable" and "risk" in detail.

Failure to appreciate how safety determinations resolve into the two discrete activities is at the root of many misunderstandings. In one of the most common instances, it gives rise to the false expectation that scientists can *measure* whether something is safe. They cannot, of course, because the methods of the physical and biological sciences can assess only the probabilities and consequences of events, not their value to people. Scientists are prepared principally to measure risks. Deciding whether people, with all their peculiarities of need, taste, tolerance, and adventurousness, might be or should be willing to bear the estimated risks is a value judgment that scientists are little better qualified to make than anyone else. Technical people such as engineers, scientists, and physicians do venture such judgments when they design an automobile or power saw, advise the government about the safety of food colorings, or prescribe an antibiotic. And social scientists, such as market researchers, poll people's attitudes toward taking certain risks. Often, though, risks are weighed by a nonscientist consumer, manufacturer, or political official: a consumer purchases a power lawn mower, a manufacturer decides whether to incorporate a safeguarding feature in one of his products, or a legislator takes a stand on automotive pollution control. Our point is not to criticize any of these actions, but rather to urge that they be recognized for what they are.

Safety is obviously a highly relative attribute that can change from time to time and be judged differently in different contexts. Knowledge of risks evolves, and so do our personal and social standards of acceptability. Our decision whether to cross a street is different on different days, depending on whether it is raining, for instance, or whether we are carrying a heavy load of groceries, or whether we are already late for an appointment. A power saw that is safe for an adult may not be safe in the hands of a child. Partly because we have discovered adverse health effects we didn't know about earlier, and partly because more sensitive techniques are now available, X-ray doses thought safe forty years ago are now deemed intolerably risky. DDT is essentially banned from most uses in the United States, where we have access to and can afford more costly alternatives, are not so much exposed to tropical diseases, and can afford to be concerned about even a slight risk of cancer—but in contrast, DDT is the pesticide of choice in many tropical, less wealthy countries where every

9

scrap of food has to be protected from insect predators, and where malaria and other diseases carried by DDT-susceptible insects are more imminent threats to life than the remote possibility of cancer.

Gauging risk is a matter of probabilities. A risk estimate can assess the overall chance that an untoward event will occur, but it is powerless to predict any specific event. From various evidence we can determine the likelihood that an automobile part will break and cause an accident; but we cannot predict *which* individual automobile will be the unlucky one or *when* the part will fail. By surveying large numbers of women we can estimate the general risk of uterine infection for users of intrauterine contraceptive devices, but we are helpless to predict which particular women will suffer that infection in the future. The great advantage of thinking in terms of probabilities is that it enables us to make broad comparisons among different hazardous circumstances. Risk is not an unfamiliar concept; it is involved at least implicitly in activities ranging from finance to romance.

In recent years safety decisions have been accorded increasing importance. New products, many of novel design, are being put on the market faster than society can test them all thoroughly for hazard. As we have become more aware of the interdependence of the parts of our environment we have tried to learn to anticipate the consequences that a change in one sector, such as agricultural pest control, will have on other sectors, such as the health of the ocean environment. The rights granted to workers are changing; a person no longer has to perform his job strictly at his own peril. Safety has become important in marketing consumer products. As people become less vulnerable to diseases and other natural hazards, the risks from manmade hazards gain importance. As we come to understand the causes of illness and injury, we worry about adverse effects, such as some genetic effects, that we weren't even aware of until a few years ago. The growth of the scale of human events has dwarfed the ability of individuals to estimate, appraise, and reduce their own risks. For all these reasons, the rational and centralized determination of safety has been gaining importance.

The public's expectation is that science and technology can and should get us out of some of the problems they got us into in the first place. From the laboratory and the factory and the agency comes the reply: Yes, much can be done to learn more and to keep us safer, and much will be done; but each aspect of the work has its costs, and society will have to decide what it wants to pay for and make the required commitment of resources.

In attempting to steer among the pitfalls we have devised for ourselves, we continually have to seek a proper balance between the comprehensive, rigorous, rational approaches that seem so essential, and the subjective, less quantifiable but not necessarily less valid approaches characteristic of political and social confrontations with the unknown. Just as the public and its political leaders must avoid irrationality, technical people must avoid illegitimate pretensions to authority. Failure to blend the several approaches satisfactorily will weaken our defenses against these unprecedented threats and will weaken the humanistic cause as well.

Since the taking of both personal and societal risks is inherent in human activity, there can be no hope of reducing all risks to zero. Rather, as when steering any course, we must continually adjust our heading so as to enjoy the greatest benefit at the lowest risk and cost. This book is about plotting courses. Its intent is not to lay out specific charts, but to describe, however flawed they may be, some of the available techniques of navigation.

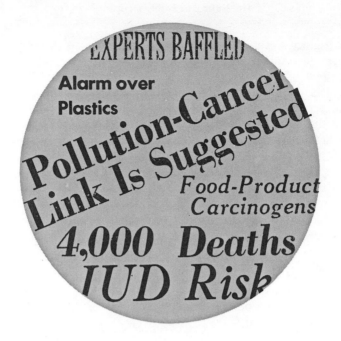

2

Measuring Risk

When the safety of a thing comes into question, whether it is a new product or an old matter newly under suspicion, the risks from exposure to it have to be measured. This chapter surveys the problems of identifying which properties are responsible for adverse effects, designing experiments to measure those effects, making the measurements, evaluating the reliability of the findings, and interpreting the evidence in sizing up the risks.

For a new problem, it is seldom sufficient just to select tests from reference books or apply on-the-shelf instruments in some standard way. The hazard usually must be scrutinized from several vantages, and new analytical techniques may have to be devised. The first, most difficult task is to select from among the many possibilities those measurements most pertinent to the problem at hand.

The purpose of measuring is to quantify, to produce numbers: the percentage of electric drills that short-circuit during extended-use tests; the temperature at which a fabric ignites; the mortality among mice exposed to chemical vapors; the degree of hearing impairment in people exposed to a noise; the incidence of cancer among workers in a factory; the amount of lead in children's blood. The task is to design the measurements so that the numbers obtained will have the greatest significance for indicating risk.

In recent years the techniques of measurement have been refined to a degree unimaginable a few decades ago. As we will illustrate shortly, these new methods often generate new data at such a rate and with such sensitivity that theory is strained to explain them. Just as the development of science can be looked upon in part as a history of improvements in technique, the development of our knowledge about hazards reflects a history of improvements in our ability to measure risk.

One of the most important tactics of research is to recognize how knowledge gained in one area can be applied to questions arising in seemingly different, but fundamentally related, areas. For example, such apparently unrelated problems as the health risks of apricot-kernel oil used as cherry flavoring, the risks to workers in a silverplating shop, the environmental risks of the western rangelands, and some of the risks of a burning office building are actually all related in that in all four cases a major toxic principle involved is cyanide (from slow deterioration of the apricot oil, from electroplating solutions, from poisons spread to kill gophers, and from high-temperature breakdown of foamed polyurethane insulation, respectively). What we learn about the hazards of the high-powered microwave devices used in transcontinental communication may apply to the much weaker microwave ovens designed for home kitchen use. Knowledge of the cancer-inducing properties of the dye industry's chemical, benzpyrene, is important for analyzing the hazards of tobacco smoke, of which benzpyrene is a constituent.

SOURCES OF EVIDENCE

Evidence regarding possible threat to health may be gathered from many sources:

- Traditional or folk knowledge
- Common-sense assessment
- Analogy to well-known cases
- Experiments on human subjects

- Review of inadvertent and occupational exposure
- Epidemiological surveys
- Experiments on nonhuman organisms
- Tests of product performance

Clearly these categories overlap. The first three are quite general; the last five are more specific and will warrant special treatment later in this chapter. We begin with an overview.

Quite often an issue has a history about which there is some *traditional or folk knowledge*. A few years ago lead was found to be leaching into some foods stored in containers coated with improperly fired lead-based glazes; this was nothing new, but was a revival of a problem known since ancient Roman times. In one illustrative case from 1967, a 55-year-old physician was hospitalized with puzzling symptoms which were eventually diagnosed, after several weeks of detective work, as those of lead poisoning. How would such a healthy and knowledgeable man become poisoned? The case was a mystery until persistent questioning finally revealed that every night for the preceding two years the man had pursued a habit of sipping a soft drink from a favorite ceramic mug made by his son in a college crafts class. In a laboratory test a mugful of the acidic cola was found to dissolve more than 5 milligrams of lead from the glaze in half an hour, a dangerously high amount.[5] This was the very same problem the Romans encountered in storing cider and wine in their lead-glazed pottery, a hazard some historians believe may have caused chronic poisoning of the aristocracy, lowering fertility and general health and contributing to the fall of the Roman Empire. Reviewing the medical report cited above, and similar ones dealing with commercial ceramics, in the light of traditional knowledge has led the Food and Drug Administration to tighten enforcement of its glazing standards. Many familiar items are traditionally known to be hazardous. We recall folk knowledge of poisonous berries, tubers, and certain mineral springs, and of elaborate methods for preserving and cooking various foods to make them safe to eat.

Sometimes a problem can be dealt with by *common-sense assessment*. In the 1960s there was some question as to the advisability of incorporating compounds called "glycerides" into such processed foods as shortening, margarine, and baked foods in order to modify texture and other physical

---

[5]Robert W. Harris and W. R. Elsea, "Ceramic glaze as a source of lead poisoning," *Journal of the American Medical Association 202,* 544-546 (1967).

properties. After study, this use was held justifiable because identical or very similar glycerides are normally present in comparable amounts in many natural, completely accepted foods. The argument went as follows. From analyses of natural foods and from surveys of people's eating habits, it was estimated that a normal diet includes as much as 30 to 50 grams of glycerides per day. The proposed glyceride additives would have added about one gram per day to an average diet. Therefore, it was reasoned, the addition of one or two grams of glycerides to the diet as additives would be only a slight increase over the natural "background" and should not present a significant new hazard.[6]

Analogy to well-known cases often provides insight. In a controversy over urban noise standards one can review such thoroughly studied problems as hearing loss among artillerymen, of which the military have made many reliable measurements. Other analogy might be found in the often cited 1965 study of the hearing of Scottish jute weavers, women who had been exposed to the slamming and roaring of the jute mills for many years, who had become partially deaf to both high- and low-frequency sounds.[7] Measurements of the urban noise at issue can provide a profile of its intensity at various frequencies, and this can be compared with the characteristics of the artillery and jute mill noises, whose effects are already known. By analogy, then, at least a rough expectation of the degree of harm can be developed.

Experiments on human subjects provide uniquely convincing evidence, because physiologically and psychologically, as well as socially, the best model for mankind will always be man. The effects of low exposures can be studied and the results extrapolated in order to estimate the effects of dangerously high exposures, for which performing the direct experiment would be unconscionable. One fervently hopes that such experiments would be conducted only under the most thoughtful ethical conditions, under close supervision by the investigators, and with full, informed, voluntary consent of the subjects. The great usefulness—and the possibility of proceeding humanely—of testing materials on human volunteers has been demonstrated repeatedly. Without such experiments much of what we now understand about drugs, pesticides, food additives, and

---

[6]National Academy of Sciences/National Research Council, Food Protection Committee, *The Safety of Monoglycerides and Diglycerides for Use as Intentional Additives in Foods,* 1965.

[7]W. Taylor, J. Pearson, and A. Mair, "Study of noise and hearing in jute weaving," *Journal of the Acoustical Society of America 38,* 113-120 (1965).

other things would still be a mystery. But there are obviously many difficulties, to which we will return.[8]

Much can be learned by *review of inadvertent and occupational exposure*. People are exposed to hazards through accident, war, and natural disaster, and those experiences can be studied to great benefit. Occupational exposure provides especially important evidence. Because workers typically experience long-term exposure at rather high intensity compared to that of the general population, investigation of their health may lead to early identification of hazards to which the rest of society is exposed at much lower levels. An added research advantage is that it is often possible, because of the close and consistent association between workers and their environment, to link effects with their causes compellingly: no one doubts that coal miners' black lung disease is caused by coal dust. Asbestos fibers provide another example; they are a serious hazard, aggravating the delicate inner lining of the lungs and causing the debilitating scarring known as *asbestosis*. Much of what we know about the effects of asbestos comes from studies of miners, processors, insulation installers, and others who are heavily exposed to the material for years. Comparing their health with that of people rarely exposed has provided insights available in no other way.[9]

Hazardous effects can be related to their causes by making *epidemiological surveys*. Although the term *epidemiological* has become familiar as a variant of the medical term, epidemic, its meaning is now taken very broadly to encompass the systematic study of things which are, literally, *epi + demos*: "upon the people." The principal technique used is statistical analysis. In this approach, a survey probes the correlation between some exposure (to asbestos, or cigarette smoke) and some effect (asbestosis, or laryngeal cancer). Historically, the technique has been the key to tracing the causes of many diseases. In the early 1800s, for instance, it was used to show that people who contracted the dread disease, rabies, had in common the misfortune of having been bitten by dogs; this of course suggested that the infective agent is transmitted in the dogs' saliva, and led to control of the disease. The techniques of epidemiology have incriminated many non-infective hazards as well. In a classic case, a 1925 survey of workers employed in the watchmaking industry showed that a surprising number were afflicted by a normally rare cancer of the jaw. It turned out

---

[8]See p. 45ff.

[9]Paul Brodeur, *The Expendable Americans* (Viking, N.Y., 1974). See p. 50ff. of this book for further discussion of inadvertent and occupational exposure.

that those affected were all women who had the job of meticulously painting the numerals on the watch dials with luminous radium paint. Further investigation revealed that the women had developed the ruinous habit of shaping their tiny brushes to a point with their lips, thereby ingesting the radioactive radium, which eventually induced the cancer.[10] More recent and perhaps more familiar examples of the epidemiological approach are the highly publicized attempts to correlate the occurrence of lung cancer with smoking cigarettes and with breathing polluted air, and to correlate occupational exposure to certain chemicals with increased incidence of normally rare tumors. Such after-the-fact investigations do not require deliberately subjecting humans to hazards, and much can be learned from them; however, they can at best only *suggest* causal relationships, which must then be confirmed in other ways.[11]

Many questions require *experiments on nonhuman organisms.* The object of *controlled experimentation* is to treat groups of similar subjects in different, carefully defined ways, maintaining close control over as many variables as possible, and analyze any difference in the outcomes. Such experimentation has come to be essential, for example, in testing pharmaceuticals and food additives before they are placed on the market. Every effort is made to minimize differences among the animals in their genetic makeup, history, diet, weight, and so on. The agent in question is administered to some of the animals and not to others; the non-exposed group—the control group—is selected and otherwise treated exactly as the exposed group is, thus providing a base against which the exposed group can be compared. The notion of a controlled experiment is intuitively simple. We all construct such experiments in our daily lives: modifying a recipe by changing just one ingredient at a time, or testing a fertilizer by comparing a treated patch of grass with one left untreated. But testing birth control pills, food colorings, and pesticides is hardly so simple.[12]

Tests of product performance during manufacture, before marketing, or after marketing, can indicate hazards and suggest remedies for them. Such testing is essential to manufacturers' development work. Product testing organizations depend on it in their rating and certification programs. Although the technical aspects can become quite complicated, the general idea is familiar; we all do it as we test our bicycle's braking

---

[10]William B. Castle, Katherine R. Drinker, and Cecil K. Drinker, "Necrosis of the jaw in workers employed in applying a luminous paint containing radium," *Journal of Industrial Hygiene 7*, 371-382 (1925).

[11]See p. 52ff.

[12]See p. 53ff.

distance, proofread a page we have typed, or check up on an old household repair.[13]

Shortly we will discuss the latter five of the above sources of evidence in more detail. But since those methods generate many different kinds of answers—often to questions not even asked—we must first have in mind the principal kinds of questions that need to be addressed.

THE FOUR LINES OF INVESTIGATION

Peeled back to their essential nature, all of the many questions about hazards, whatever they specifically happen to be, divide into four lines of investigation. In assessing risk, measurements are made in order to:

1. Define the conditions of exposure;
2. Identify the adverse effects;
3. Relate exposure with effect;
4. Estimate overall risk.

These need not be sequential, although progress on one often spurs action on another. They can be pursued independently and simultaneously, but they overlap and are quite interdependent.

Defining the Conditions of Exposure

Who will be exposed? To what? In what way? For how long? Intensely for only a moment, or at a low level for a long time?

And how much hazardous agent is there? If a chemical, how concentrated? If radiation, how strong, and of what characteristics? If a hot surface, how hot? If noise, how loud?

Finding out who is at risk may not be easy. In the case of air pollution, for example, once a pollutant has left its source, predicting its dispersal is subject to all the familiar uncertainties of predicting the weather. On some days pollution may be pocketed in stale air. On other days the skies will be swept clear by the wind. The best we can do is measure conditions on a number of days, calculate averages, and estimate the variability in conditions. Then: who breathes the air? There are children and adults and the elderly, and asthmatics, and pregnant women, and people with weakened hearts. ... Again, we must deal with dissatisfyingly uncertain averages in

---

[13]See p. 55ff.

programs concerned with the composition of complex mixtures. Micro-chemical analysis was developed in the search for antimalarial drugs and other important chemicals. Spectroscopy, a fundamental research tool of both physics and chemistry, was adapted for routine analysis. What these highly refined tools began to reveal was that many things were not so free from hazard as we had always thought. But it was hard to be sure.

The controversy over DDT in recent years arose in part simply because we became able to detect the chemical with unprecedented sensitivity. Had we not, in the early 1950s, begun detecting DDT everywhere—on the ice caps, in polar bear fat, in tropical fish, in mothers' milk all over the world—we would probably not have begun to worry as we did about what it might be doing to living things. However minuscule the trace of DDT was, and however tenuous the indictment against it was, DDT nevertheless was unarguably, inescapably *there*—something to worry about.

The concentration of a substance in a mixture can be expressed in terms of parts of the chemical relative to some number of parts of all other substances. For example, one ounce of a chemical in a thousand ounces of a total mixture is said to be present at one part per thousand. By mid-century we had become able to detect chemicals, in some cases, at the level of one part per million, a much-heralded accomplishment. In 1951, DDT was detected in human milk at one-tenth of one part per million.[16]

To envision a part per million, consider a jar of sugar into which a single crystal of table salt has been dropped. A crystal of salt weighs about one-tenth of a milligram. Therefore, if a one-hundred-gram (four-ounce) jar of sugar has a single grain of salt dropped into it, the mixture contains salt at about one part per million. One speck of salt in half a cup of sugar: one part per million. In recent years the limits of detection have been pushed down so far that it has become necessary to introduce the term *parts per billion*—and now there is even reference to parts per trillion, an amount a million times less concentrated than a part per million.[17]

One controversy after another has pivoted upon very small amounts of chemicals contaminating our food or environment: the weed killer amino-triazole detected in the 1959 cranberry crop at a few parts per million; a

---

[16]Edwin P. Laug, Frieda M. Kunze, and C. S. Prickett, "Occurrence of DDT in human fat and milk," *American Medical Association, Archives of Industrial Hygiene and Occupational Medicine 3*, 245-246 (1951). For the history of DDT, see Chapter 6.

[17]Donald J. Lisk, "Recent developments in the analysis of toxic elements," *Science 184*, 1137-1141 (1974).

part per million of mercury in tuna; the synthetic chemicals called poly-chlorinated biphenyls (PCBs) found in the waters of the North Atlantic at approximately twenty parts per trillion; and dioxin, the exceedingly toxic impurity in the weedkiller, 2,4,5-T, found in some parts of the environment at a part or so per trillion.

But is a part per billion or trillion of anything worth worrying about? The answer is different for different substances, and the rationale differs from case to case, as examples later in this book will illustrate. There is no doubt that some substances affect organisms even at extraordinarily low levels. Because of its toxicity, mercury is usually not considered acceptable in the diet at levels greater than fifty parts per billion.[18] Plutonium, which must be handled daily by the nuclear industry, is extremely toxic to animals and probably also to man.[19] And about one ten-billionth of a gram of *botulinus* poison is enough to kill a mouse.[20]

The general point is that a peculiar concern arises when contaminating trace substances are detected: even if harmful effects are merely suspected and not yet proven, once a contaminant is known to be in food or in the environment its presence cannot be ignored. This anxiety may stem at least partly from revulsion against polluting our very own flesh; an uneasy feeling comes over us when we learn that DDT, the active ingredient of lice spray, taints the milk of every mother on earth. Our sophistication in detecting and identifying the most minuscule traces of chemicals, no matter where they occur, has forced us to change our fundamental notions about presence and absence of chemicals.

In virtually everything, there now seems to be at least a little bit of everything else. This is especially true of substances that are both chemically stable and physically mobile. This realization has given rise to a host of new worries. Some turn out to be false. But others prove to be legitimate and worthy of serious attention.

Similar advances in detection have occurred in other fields besides chemistry. Radiation detection has improved. We are much better able to analyze noise. The statistical techniques of epidemiology and of the social sciences have been refined. Biologists now have powerful electron micro-scopes capable of magnifying things to a million times their actual size.

---

[18]World Health Organization/Food and Agriculture Organization/International Atomic Energy Agency International Discussion, "Mercury contamination of man and his environment," 1967.

[19]Medical Research Council, United Kingdom, *The Toxicity of Plutonium* (Her Majesty's Stationery Office, London, 1975).

[20]Carl Lamanna, "The most poisonous poison," *Science 130*, 763-772 (1959).

When the municipal drinking water of Duluth, Minnesota, which appears clear and free of particulate matter under an ordinary light microscope, was examined in 1973 with such an electron microscope, it was found to contain up to a hundred billion tiny fibers of asbestos in every liter. Should we worry? Heavy feeding tests with dogs have shown that asbestos in this form can give the dogs cancer. It is not clear whether humans are affected similarly. Should an effort be made to remove the asbestos, present for years but never before even detected, from Duluth's water? Should the mining company that has been discharging its mine wastes into Lake Superior, the source of the water, be required to take expensive corrective action? At this writing scientific studies and legal action continue. The case will set important precedents on the issue of who bears the burden of proof and whether actual damage to human health has to be demonstrated before courts can take action. Again, simply detecting the material is what touched off a debate with broad medical, economic, and legal implications.[21]

Identifying the Adverse Effects

Having some idea of who is exposed, and to what, allows us to move on and ask, "What's the threat?" Is the appliance likely to deliver an electric shock, or does its casing get so hot that people can burn themselves on it? This pesticide is lethal to insects; is its effect on humans that of a general poison, or might it be carcinogenic? In planning to use this chemical as an industrial intermediate, should we protect against allergenic reaction, against fire hazard, or what? If we fluoridate our water, which health effects should we monitor for?

Such questions may not be amenable to systematic pursuit. In fact, they often arise in an inverse way: an accident occurs, or dead fish wash up on shore, or isolated reports of an unusual tumor begin to form a pattern and suggest that a new problem is arising. Looking back over safety controversies with benefit of hindsight reveals that the more subtle ill effects may not be recognized until the situation becomes rather aggravated. Often this is because the questions have been asked not in the form, "What effects will this thing have?" but rather, "What caused these undesirable events?" Similarities among isolated events may not become evident for a long time.

---

[21]"Pollution and public health: Taconite case poses major test," *Science 186*, 31-36 (1974).

Hazards may be revealed through investigation of accidents and illnesses, through systematic testing of products, or through epidemiological surveys. Sometimes a fundamental scientific advance reveals a mechanism of hazard not even suspected before, as in the following example of biological damage due to X-rays.

Around the turn of the century, when X-rays were first being used in medicine, these marvelous beams that could penetrate solid objects were the subject of great curiosity. People had themselves X-rayed just for fun. Physicians performed experiments on themselves, and their findings held great promise. The technique was going to be a boon to medicine. The principal side effect recognized was a seemingly unimportant irritation, or burning, of the skin. In the earliest days physicians even used this effect to test the strength of the radiation beam by passing their hands through the beam and observing the reddening, or erythema, of the backs of their hands (more reddening indicated that the beam was stronger). Reports of serious erythema among both physicians and patients accumulated; the medical literature of the period carried many references to this hazard.[22] The early X-ray experiments caused so much grief that a memorial honor roll, *American Martyrs to Science Through the Roentgen Rays,* was published.[23] Not until 1927, when H. J. Muller discovered by experimenting with fruit flies that X-rays could damage chromosomes, was there evidence of a threat to inheritance. That discovery drastically changed the complexion of the problem. Although erythema still had to be contended with, the problem of genetic hazard is much more elusive, more disturbing, and in the long run more significant to the human race. In the 1950s, another adverse effect of radiation was confirmed when it became clear that the survivors of the Hiroshima and Nagasaki explosions were afflicted with leukemia to an unusual degree. Other health effects have been discovered since then. This important twentieth-century example makes it clear that even with all the care and attention given to major innovations, adverse effects may pass undetected for many years.

From our everyday experience we are only too familiar with different modes of injury. *Mechanical injuries*—cuts, bruises, abrasions, broken bones, and so forth—take an enormous toll. The damage is usually

---

[22]Barbara Spencer Marx, *Early experiences with the hazards of medical use of X-rays: 1896-1906,* George Washington University; National Technical Information Service PB 182877 (1968); M. K. Kassabian, *Roentgen Rays and Electro-Therapeutics* (Lippincott, Philadelphia, 1910).

[23]Percy Brown, *American Martyrs to Science through the Roentgen Rays* (C. C. Thomas, Springfield, Illinois, 1936).

obvious at once. But sometimes the effects are slow to develop, as when a person's hearing is gradually impaired by repetitive and cumulative mechanical damage to the delicate apparatus of his ears by loud noises, or when jarring vibrations slowly induce back injury in an operator of heavy mechanical equipment.

Burn is another common injury. It can range from a nuisance endured perennially in preparing meals to a horrible fatal accident in handling industrial solvents. Its primary effects are evident immediately.

Electrical shock is instantaneous and may range in seriousness from an annoyance to a fatality. Although electrical accidents are often caused by user negligence, this is one hazard from which we expect to be responsibly protected by sound product design.

Chemical poisoning is an inconveniently broad term, but we will use it to mean physiological damage caused by a chemical. The effect may be immediate, as when a child swallows lye or cleaning fluid, or it may be a longer-term effect, as with gradual liver damage to an industrial worker who breathes a solvent-laden atmosphere day after day in the course of his work.

Irritation and sensitization are very common problems. We all know people who suffer the agonies of allergy to pollens, feathers, poison ivy, and insect stings. The Public Health Service reports that "hundreds of thousands of workers each year suffer skin diseases from contact with materials from their work. The dermatoses are the most common of all occupational illnesses."[24] The smog that hovers over urban areas causes reactions ranging from eye irritation to asthmatic crisis, and rather serious reactions can arise to everyday materials such as soaps, detergents, cleaning fluids, and cosmetics. Signs of effect may not show up at first, making the search for the guilty agent difficult. Irritants can be distinguished from allergens: *irritants* (such as shampoo in the eye) elicit reaction from most people almost immediately upon contact, but the effect is temporary and subsequent similar exposures are no more harmful. *Allergens* (such as poison ivy) affect different people in different ways, harming only those who have become sensitized to the allergen. Sensitization can build up over days or months as a person is exposed; then, without warning, in the course of a familiar routine activity, as the substance is handled one more time, reaction erupts. A rash breaks out, or a scale develops on the skin, or eyes begin to itch, and from then on the person is afflicted with what can be a miserable malady. In some

---

[24]U. S. Department of Health, Education, and Welfare, "Occupational Disease . . . The silent enemy."

cases dermal reactions called photosensitization reactions are caused by chemicals and sunlight working in concert, as occasionally happens when a lipstick is worn at the beach.

The kinds of injury listed above are rather easily detected; for the most part, their symptoms become evident fairly soon after exposure. Effects can usually be connected to their causes. But there are other adverse effects which are much more difficult to detect and assess.

Carcinogenesis is the induction of runaway growth of the cells of some part of the body. The resulting disease condition, commonly referred to by the broad term *cancer*, can take many forms. Despite several decades of intensive worldwide effort to understand the causes of cancer and to develop remedies, we still know disappointingly little. The problem is of enormous scope, and the campaign against cancer carries a strong sense of urgency. Thousands of research workers in industrial, university, medical center, and government laboratories are devoted to the search for causes and cures. Through the years a series of congressional acts has committed more than three billion dollars to the attack on cancer. The National Cancer Institute estimates that during 1973 in the United States 350,000 people died of cancer and 665,000 new cases were diagnosed; at this rate, more than 53,000,000 Americans now living—one-fifth of the entire population—are expected to develop some kind of cancer eventually.[25]

The agents known to cause cancer are many and varied; they include chemicals, viruses, radiation, and particulate matter. Protracted exposure of workers to certain industrial chemicals can induce cancer of the lungs. The increased incidence of leukemia, a blood cancer, among survivors of the Nagasaki and Hiroshima atomic bomb explosions attests to the carcinogenic properties of radiation. An unusually large number of farmers and fishermen develop cancer of the neck and lip from long exposure to direct sunlight. The thorough, highly publicized reports of the U.S. Surgeon General implicate cigarette smoke in causing several kinds of cancer.

The diversity of the agents causing cancer, and the multiplicity of forms in which the disease may be manifested, calls for an operational definition something like the following: "For practical purposes, a carcinogen is a substance that when administered by an appropriate route, causes an increased incidence of malignant tumors in experimental animals as

---

[25]*National Cancer Institute Fact Book 1973,* U. S. National Institutes of Health Publication No. 73-512 (1973).

26

compared with a control series of untreated animals."[26] Many current safety debates—cyclamates, radiation, vinyl chloride, the pesticides dieldrin and aldrin—center in part upon whether the agents are carcinogenic.[27]

Mutagenesis, modification of the body's genetic material, has been of public concern since the discovery that X-rays are mutagenic. That concern increased when it was found that various chemicals and ultraviolet light also could cause genetic alteration. And then, with the release of the mutation-inducing atomic genie in the 1940s, the problem of mutagenesis became a major burden on the conscience of mankind. As one advisory panel so aptly said, "Surely one of the greatest responsibilities of our generation is our temporary custody of the genetic heritage received from our ancestors. We must make every reasonable effort to insure that this heritage is passed on to future generations undamaged. To do less, we believe, is grossly irresponsible."[28]

Teratogenesis is alteration of the development of a baby in the womb, causing it to be born deformed or defective. Although a lot of research and therapeutic attention had been given to the problem of birth defects, it was not until the thalidomide disaster of the early 1960s that teratogenesis commanded much government attention.[29] The public became aware that birth defects don't "just happen," but are caused by specific agents. The 1963 President's Science Advisory Committee report, *Use of Pesticides*, was one of the first major studies to recommend that chemicals such as pesticides be routinely tested for teratogenicity before being placed on the market.[30]

Although *behavioral impairment* may be difficult to detect and analyze, it can nevertheless be an important effect of otherwise apparently mild hazards, such as noise. Except for rather obvious cases such as alcoholism or side effects of pharmaceuticals, few low-level hazards have been

---

[26]Food and Drug Administration Advisory Committee on Protocols for Safety Evaluation, "Panel on Carcinogenesis Report on Cancer Testing in the Safety Evaluation of Food Additives and Pesticides," *Toxicology and Applied Pharmacology 20,* 419 (1971).

[27]John Cairns, "The cancer problem," *Scientific American 233,* No. 5, 64-78 (1975).

[28]U. S. Department of Health, Education, and Welfare, *Report of the HEW Secretary's Commission on Pesticides and Their Relationship to Environmental Health,* 568 (1969); for a good general discussion see Alexander Hollaender, *Chemical Mutagens* (Plenum, New York, 1971), and the Environmental Mutagen Society, committee 17, "Environmental Mutagenic Hazards," *Science 187,* 503-514 (1975).

[29]H. Sjöström and R. Nilsson, *Thalidomide and the Power of the Drug Companies* (Penguin, Harmondsworth, England, 1972).

[30]President's Science Advisory Committee, *Use of Pesticides,* 21 (1963).

proven to have strong effects on human behavior. But incriminating evidence is building up.[31] To cite an example that is often mentioned, many pesticides exert their toxic action on insects by attacking the nervous system; it is not clear whether at extremely low doses, such as those passed on to humans in the food chain, there is a corresponding but subtle effect on human beings.

No one disagrees that noise interferes with conversation, mental concentration, and sleep. It impairs hearing. But does noise ever cause more permanent mental disorders? The evidence is inconclusive. Mental illness, nausea, and general anxiety have all been attributed to noise, but "these effects are difficult to assess because intense noises are often associated with situations that in and of themselves, even without noise, might involve fear and stress. Whether the noise, purely as noise, contributes significantly to the stress of life ... is difficult to assess at this time."[32]

Each of the above problems commands the attention of many research workers and is the subject of an extensive literature. Our few paragraphs could only identify some of the terms so we can refer to them as we proceed.[33]

Identifying adverse effects is more difficult than one might think. There are major problems, of course, in doing laboratory analyses, making medical diagnoses, determining behavioral effects, studying accident patterns, and assembling statistics. But these are mostly technical problems, and they can be solved. But knowing what to look for is a different matter; failure to anticipate and search appropriately for adverse effects is the cause of many public surprises. It was only after the enzyme-containing detergents had been hastily developed, tested, and rushed onto the market as successors to the ecologically offending phosphates a few years ago that the possibility of skin sensitization began to be considered widely. Currently, the United States is on the verge of adopting catalytic converter devices for automobiles in order to reduce the emission of pollutants; but one cannot help wondering whether some of the adverse effects of these devices, such as the release of sulfuric acid and metallic

---

[31]B. Weiss and V. G. Laties, "Behavioral pharmacology and toxicology," *Annual Review of Pharmacology 9*, 297-326 (1969).

[32]U. S. Environmental Protection Agency, *Effects of Noise on People,* 123 (1971).

[33]Excellent description of many modes of injury can be found in the World Health Organization's *Health Hazards of the Human Environment* (Geneva, 1972).

compounds into the air, have been adequately anticipated and appraised.[34] During a crash program to remedy some technological threat it is easy to overlook side effects; but the sad consequence may be that the old problem is simply replaced by new ones that are even less well understood.

Relating Exposure with Effect

Now we turn to the problem of relating exposure with effect, dose with response, use with result. Here we move from "*What* are the adverse effects?" to "*How much* adverse effect results from *how much* exposure?"

Although the concept underlying this step is intuitively straightforward—if a little bit causes a little effect, more should cause a larger effect, and a lot should cause a very large effect—the actual business of quantifying the relationship can be quite complicated. This line of investigation is often the most difficult one for scientists in the laboratory.

The objective of this step is to make the sort of correlation depicted in Figure 2-1. The axes of the graph represent the outcomes of the first two lines of investigation: the conditions of exposure (abscissa) and the resultant adverse effects (ordinate). One may be plotting quite specific effects, such as increase in blood pressure from various dosages of a drug, or general effects, such as clinical signs of lead poisoning relative to amount of lead ingested.

Lead poisoning provides a good illustration. Lead, a relatively abundant, soft, workable metal, has been used through the ages to make eating and drinking vessels, plumbing, printing type, and many other common items. Its largest use at present is in storage batteries. Alloyed with other low-melting metals it forms the most commonly used solders. In the form of pewter, its alloy with tin, it was long used to make lovely household objects (but notice that modern pewter should not contain lead). White lead oxide and red lead oxide are still widely used in industrial paints; tetraethyl lead is the common antiknock additive in gasoline; and other lead compounds are used in glazes for ceramics. In all these forms lead is a poison. The public health hazards are familiar: people are poisoned by drinking from old lead-based pewter mugs, children become ill from eating flakes of old paint off walls, and we all breathe pollution from automobiles burning leaded fuel.

---

[34]Arthur J. Magida, "EPA study may bring reprieve for catalytic converter," *National Journal Reports,* 552-558 (April 12, 1975).

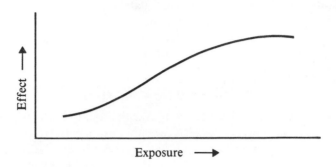

Figure 2-1. Generalized exposure-effect correlation.

Suppose one needs to relate exposure to effect. The first line of investigation shows that lead is present at certain levels—so many parts per million in the air of a city, or so many micrograms per 100 grams of factory workers' blood. The second line of investigation reveals the adverse effects and their clinical indicators: that among many other signs, for instance, a reliable indicator of lead poisoning is decrease in blood level of the enzyme, delta-aminolevulinic acid dehydrase (abbreviated ALAD; for illustrative purposes it isn't necessary to understand how the enzyme works, other than to recognize that lead poisoning diminishes the amount of ALAD in the blood). A study like that done by Sven Hernberg and his colleagues at the University of Helsinki might be carried out.[35] They measured the indicator enzyme ALAD in four groups of persons having different exposures to lead: medical students, who presumably are not much exposed; workers in printshops, who handle type metal; automobile repair workers, who work with lead batteries and solder; and lead smelters and shipscrappers, who, in refining the metal and cutting junked ships apart, respectively, can hardly avoid exposure to the metal and its fumes. The exposure-effect correlation in Figure 2-2 plots the effect, ALAD depression, against the concentration of lead in the blood, an index of exposure. (Note that other clinical studies have already established that lowering ALAD levels has an adverse effect on health.) Clearly, the more people are exposed, the higher their blood lead becomes and the more their ALAD is depressed. Individuals' responses vary, but

[35]Sven Hernberg, Jorma Nikkanen, Guy Mellin, and Helena Lilius, "δ-Aminolevulinic acid dehydrase as a measure of lead exposure," *Archives of Environmental Health 21*, 140-145 (1970).

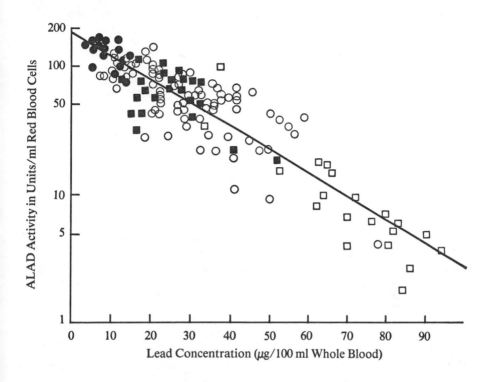

Figure 2-2. Correlation between ALAD activity and blood lead concentration for 158 persons having different exposures to lead.*

the trend is clear and average responses can be estimated. The above correlation is only one aspect of the problem, but it fits with all the other pieces of experimental and clinical evidence to build an overall picture, such as that presented in Figure 2-3, from a recent review.[36]

[36]National Academy of Sciences/National Research Council, Committee on Biologic Effects of Air Pollutants, *Lead,* 107 (1972).

*From Sven Hernberg et al., "δ-Aminolevulinic acid dehydrase as a measure of lead exposure," Archives of Environmental Health 21, 140-148 (1970).

Relating exposure to effect as illustrated above helps in diagnosing cases of lead poisoning, setting standards for exposure, and designing further studies of lead poisoning.[37]

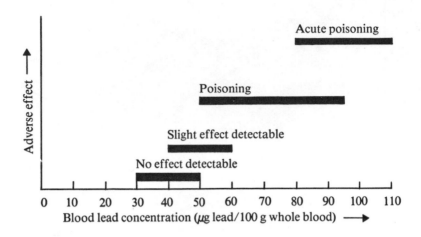

Figure 2-3. Correlation of blood lead with adverse effect.*

Quantitative correlations of effect with exposure have broad applicability to many different circumstances to exposure. Interpreted with judgment, the correlations for lead apply to every person who has lead in his blood, whether he is a junkyard worker who has to burn old lead storage batteries, or a college student ill from moonshine whiskey distilled through a lead-soldered automobile radiator. No matter what the mode of exposure, if the person's blood level is greater than 40 to 50 micrograms (μg) of lead per hundred grams of blood (see Figure 2-3), he is likely to be suffering at least mild lead poisoning. Medical supervision and further surveillance of his health are called for, and investigation of the circumstances may reveal other people under similar risk.

With regard to chemicals which are quite toxic and which are likely to be encountered intensely over a very short period (acutely), there is a classic measure of general toxicity. Referred to as the *median lethal dose* (abbreviated LD_{50}), it is defined as that dose of a substance which is

---

[37]J. Julian Chisolm, Jr., "Lead poisoning," *Scientific American 224*, 15-23 (February, 1971).

*Adapted from National Academy of Sciences/National Research Council, *Lead*, 128-129 (1972).

sufficient to kill one-half of a specified group of animals. Estimates of lethal doses can be made for man. Obviously, the smaller the LD_{50}, the more toxic the substance is, since less of the chemical is required for lethal effect. Table 2-1 lists rat LD_{50}'s for a few common compounds, in order of decreasing toxicity. The problems of defining and measuring the lethal dose for various substances form part of the professional practice of toxicology and need not concern us here.[38]

Table 2-1.   Median Lethal Doses (LD_{50}'s) of several common substances (administered orally to rats).*

Compound	LD_{50} (milligrams of compound per kilogram rat body weight)
potassium cyanide	10
tetraethyl lead	35
lead	100
DDT	150
phenobarbital	660
aspirin	1500
table salt	3000

*Selected from U.S. Department of Health, Education, and Welfare, Herbert E. Christensen, editor, *The Toxic Substances List,* 1973 edition.

Table 2-1 was assembled simply to illustrate the principle. The LD_{50} relates only to short-term exposure and is otherwise only crudely indicative of the effects of chronic or long-term exposure to small amounts. Chronic toxicities are not necessarily related to acute toxicities; clearly, it is possible for a compound such as lead or asbestos to have only a moderate LD_{50} but nevertheless to work in insidious ways over a long period and cause serious damage to health.

To illustrate the correlation of exposure with effect in a quite different area, let us consider the problem of noise, a nuisance and hazard with which we are only too familiar but which is just beginning to receive serious attention. A recent report estimated that "the number of workers in the U.S. exposed to noise potentially hazardous to hearing is in excess of six million and may be as high as 16 million."[39] That report estimated

[38]A standard text is T. A. Loomis, *Essentials of Toxicology* (Lea and Febiger, Philadelphia, 1968).

[39]U. S. Environmental Protection Agency, *Report to the President and Congress on Noise* (1972).

that more than 2,750,000 Americans have already suffered noise-associated hearing loss. Modern homes, with their noisy kitchen appliances, stereos, televisions, toys, and shop and yard tools, can be surprisingly hazardous to hearing; so can recreational activities such as motorboating, hunting, target shooting, and snowmobiling.

Impairment of hearing is its best substantiated effect, but noise also interferes with speech, mental concentration, and general sense of well-being. It may even contribute to the general stress of life sufficiently to weaken the body's defenses against emotional shock, fatigue, infection, and disease.[40]

The intensity, or loudness, of sound is measured on a logarithmic scale in units of decibels (abbreviated dB). The human ear, however, does not respond equally to sounds of different frequencies. Therefore, for many purposes, in order to represent with a single number the loudness of a sound composed of many frequencies, an appropriately weighted measure adjusted for the ear's response is used; the unit commonly used is the dBA, or "A-weighted" decibel. Figure 2-4 indicates some typical noise levels.

A familiar, annoying effect of noise is its interference with conversation. The effect can be displayed as in Figure 2-5 to show how, as interfering background noise increases, the distance at which communication is possible decreases. Following the 10-foot line of the graph, we see that communication is easy until the noise increases to about 57 dBA; it is possible with raised voices over interference up to 74 dBA; it is still possible, by shouting, through noise up to 93 dBA; and it is impossible beyond that.[41]

Most of us have submitted from time to time to audiometric evaluation of our hearing, in which the subject listens for the sounding of very slight tones. The minimum loudness at which a tone can be detected is called the auditory threshold for sound at that frequency, and a person's shift to a louder minimum tone as his hearing becomes impaired is referred to as a *threshold shift*. Many measurements of this sort have been made for people exposed to noise over long periods. From these studies the loss of hearing (as indicated by hearing threshold shifts) can be charted over a course of years. Shown in Figure 2-6 are the results of a survey of three

---

[40]U.S. Environmental Protection Agency, *Effects of Noise on People* (1971); Theodore Berland, *The Fight for Quiet* (Prentice-Hall, Inc., Englewood Cliffs, N. J., 1970).

[41]U. S. Environmental Protection Agency, *Effects of Noise on People,* 50 (1971).

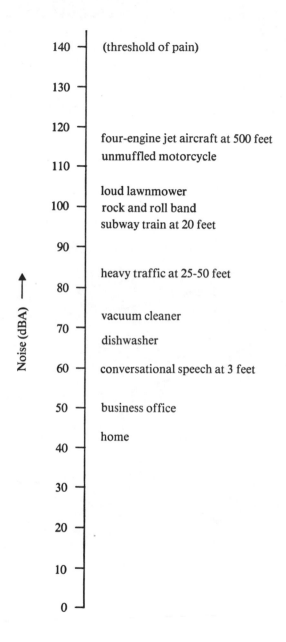

Figure 2-4. Typical noise levels.

groups of workers exposed to 83 dBA, 92 dBA, and 97 dBA continuously during their work.[42]

Measurements such as these are the basis for monitoring exposure to noise in urban, military, and occupational environments, for setting standards, and for designing quieter products. As with any such problem, technical complications arise in designing detection equipment, agreeing on standard methods for measuring, recording, and analyzing the sound, correcting for loss of hearing due to the natural processes of aging and

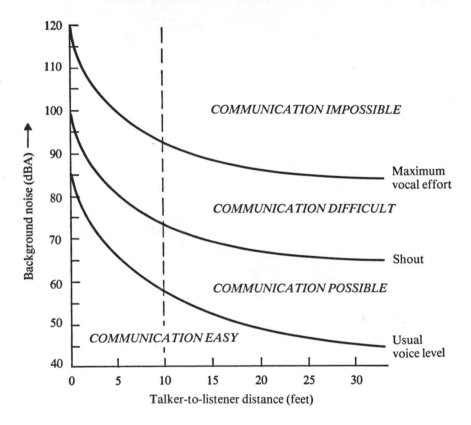

Figure 2-5.   Noise interference with speech communication, at various distances.*

[42]J. C. Nixon and A. Glorig, "Noise-induced permanent threshold shift at 2000 cps and 4000 cps," *Journal of the Acoustical Society of America 33,* 904-908 (1961).

*Adapted from U.S. Environmental Protection Agency, *Effects of Noise on People,* 50 (1971).

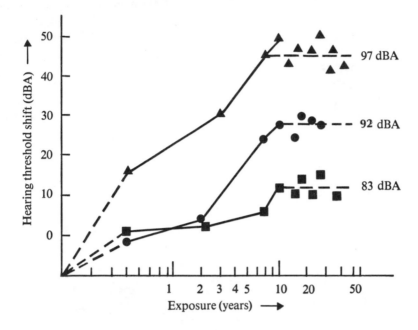

Figure 2-6. Impairment of hearing among workers exposed to 83, 92, and 97 dBA, as evidenced by permanent hearing threshold shifts (measured at 4000 Hertz, corrected for effects of aging).*

disease, and in proving that the effects can indeed be attributed to noise and not to some other environmental condition that accompanies the noise.

One can think of many more such examples, all seemingly different but actually having the same purpose: for an oral contraceptive, relating dose to occurrence of unusual bleeding; for an air pollutant, relating the incidence of eye irritations to various concentrations of pollutant.

Because correlations of exposure with effect can only be *composites of averages,* their precision is limited by our ability to subject highly non-uniform human beings to statistical scrutiny. All measurements suffer some uncertainty. In general, observations of strong, immediate effects carry more certainty than observations of subtle, delayed, less acute

*Adapted from J. C. Nixon and A. Glorig, "Noise-induced permanent threshold shift at 2000 cps and 4000 cps," Journal of the Acoustical Society of America 33, 904-908 (1961).

effects. This can be visualized in a simplified manner as in Figure 2-7, in which relations having greater uncertainty are indicated by circles of greater diameter. (In analyzing any real hazard, such an idealized curve would be resolved into several more precise curves for low exposures, high exposures, different kinds of effect, and so on.)

A number of factors account for the imprecision at the extremes of the curve. Measuring techniques have their intrinsic limits. Each individual's vulnerability varies from day to day, and physiologies vary from person to person. At very low exposures, effects may be only marginally detectable, the presence of the offending agent may be difficult to gauge, and the relation of cause to effect may be hard to prove. At the other extreme, the upper end of the curve may remain in doubt because accidental exposures are rare and because ethical considerations prohibit deliberately exposing human beings to large doses of the hazard. Extrapolating animal test findings to estimate human experience is always and unavoidably imprecise.

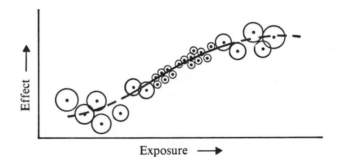

Figure 2-7.　Generalized exposure-effect curve, showing uncertainty at high and low exposures: diameter of circles indicates degree of certainty about data points.

The principal use of these curves is to predict effects at very low and very high extremes of exposure, where direct experiments cannot be made satisfactorily. Suppose the hypothetical curve shown in Figure 2-8 represents some agent's effect on humans. Animal studies and accidental poisonings have shown that amount A can be lethal, thus fixing the high end of the curve. The effects of fairly large amounts (the section from B to A) are known from accidental exposures, studies of occupationally exposed workers, and from human feeding experiments. For small amounts (less than B), there is less certainty in the plot because of difficulties in proving cause-effect relations in this range.

38

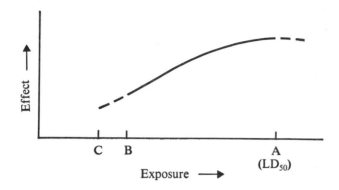

Figure 2-8. Generalized exposure-effect curve, showing three ranges of exposure and effect.

In a real situation we would likely want to ask, "What is the effect of very small amounts, such as C, the routine or occasional exposure?" Obviously we must extrapolate—but is that portion of the curve a straight line, or is it convex or concave?

Until the curve can be defined better in the low range, the best we can do is apply experience from related extrapolations and sketch in an extension such as the dotted line in Figure 2-9. The line may or may not be expected to pass through the graph's origin. The lowest normal exposure may be irreducible below some natural background. For mercury, or noise, for instance, there is always some of the element in the environment (some lower point D). Similarly, for radiation there is always a background from rocks and cosmic rays. There may be a normal background of effect as well, such as a normal minimum blood pressure.

An important concern for any agent is whether it has a *threshold* for onset of action. For example, a heat source, such as the surface of a household appliance, at around room temperature will not burn one's skin no matter how long the exposure. Increasing the temperature has no deleterious effect until a threshold is reached at about 65°C, where pain is felt. At temperatures higher than this the skin is burned with rapidly increasing severity. There is a threshold of pain, a threshold of remediable injury, and a threshold of irreversible, tissue-destroying burn. For exposure to very loud noises there is a definable threshold of pain, just as there is a much lower threshold for perception of sound. Many everyday phenomena have threshold effects. Their exposure-effect curves resemble the plot in Figure 2-10.

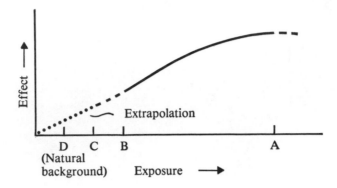

Figure 2-9.   Generalized exposure-effect curve, showing extrapolation to low levels.

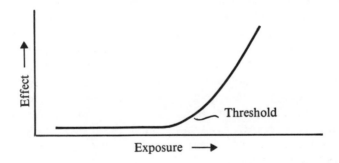

Figure 2-10. Generalized exposure-effect curve, showing threshold effect.

The phenomena of thresholds are of much more than academic interest. If it can be proven compellingly that an agent has a threshold for effect—a threshold below which the human body can take care of itself through its marvelous self-cleansing and repair mechanisms—the problem of determining safe doses and setting standards is greatly simplified. The threshold is a benchmark below which exposures carry only minimal risk. Unfortunately, there is still uncertainty; this is because people's thresholds vary, as is obvious from the simple examples of skin burn and hearing impairment. Just knowing a few individuals' thresholds

40

of susceptibility may not provide sufficient basis for establishing standards for an entire society.

Worse yet, for most toxic chemicals, radiation, and other low-level and delayed-effect hazards, the threshold question has never been satisfactorily resolved. Conflicting opinions abound. The issue of thresholds has been critical in the setting of standards for such highly contended menaces as radiation and automobile emissions. Some researchers conclude that there is indeed a threshold for teratogenic action, or carcinogenic action, or mutagenic action, while others are skeptical and urge a more cautious stance.

Estimating Overall Risk

This is the payoff stage, building upon all the preceding inquiries: the conditions of exposure having been defined and the adverse effects identified, and exposure having been related to effect, here the various consequences of exposure are summarized to yield overall estimates of risk, both to individuals and to society as a whole.

The several effects are compared in order to identify which are the strongest, the most undesirable, and the most likely to affect many people. This judgment edges up to being political as well as scientific, and its outcome often becomes the principal input to the heavily value-laden public tasks of judging the acceptability of risks and setting standards, regulating the market, planning research, and otherwise managing the hazard as a public problem.

A procedurally sound example of such an estimation is the National Research Council's 1972 study of *The Effects on Populations of Exposure to Low Levels of Ionizing Radiation*. The committee began by making the following points about the risks from radiation: (1) manmade radiation is not substantively different from radiation emanating from natural sources; (2) illnesses induced by manmade radiation are not generally different in kind from diseases having "natural" causes; (3) among the several effects of radiation, the genetic ones demand special attention because of their importance to our descendents; and (4) the total amount of genetically significant radiation currently received by the average person from manmade sources is not quite as much as the amount received from natural sources.

Having narrowed the scope of the problem by substantiating that set of basic statements, which are critical for all succeeding discussion, the report then built its risk analysis. It reviewed the various sources of genetically significant radiation (radiation which can affect heredity) and estimated the exposure of an average person, as summarized in Table 2-2.

41

Table 2-2.   Inventory of radiation received by average persons.[43]

Source	Radiation to whole body, millirem/year*	Genetically significant radiation, millirem/year*
Natural radiation		
Cosmic rays	44	
Bodily constituents	18	
Other	40	
	102 Total	90 Total
Man-made radiation		
Medical and dental	73	
Fallout	4	
Occupational	0.3	
Nuclear power (1970)	0.003	
	78 Total	30-60 Total

*The millirem is a measure of biologically important radiation received by a person.

The report then reviewed the adverse effects of radiation, some of which are genetic and some somatic (affecting the body in a nonheritable way). It prefaced its catalogue of genetic effects by saying that whether caused by radiation or by other well-known mutagens, "some results of genetic change are conspicuous, others are invisible; some are tragic, others so mild as to be trivial; some occur in the first generation following the gene or chromosome change, others are postponed tens or hundreds of generations into the future." It estimated genetic risk, and it summarized the difficulties of arriving at precise figures. It listed the many somatic effects of radiation, including growth impairment, mental retardation, cataracting of the lens, sterilization, and induction of cancers of the thyroid, bone, skin, breast, lung, and white blood cells.

Using all the information outlined above (which represent the first three lines of investigation in our scheme), the report then estimated overall risk to the human population from radiation, expressing that risk in four ways: "(a) risk relative to natural background radiation ... (b) risk estimates for specific genetic conditions ... (c) risk relative to current prevalence of serious disabilities ... and (d) the risk in terms of overall ill-health."

The above analysis pursued all four of our lines of investigation: it defined the conditions of exposure, detailing who is exposed to how much of what kind of radiation and comparing the contributions from various sources; it identified the adverse effects on health, both genetic and somatic; it related exposure to effect; and then, on those bases, it estimated the overall risks.

Addressing itself principally to the scientific business of estimating risk, the study did not endorse any specific exposure standards, leaving that to regulatory bodies. Its task was to "review the scientific bases used for the evaluation of risks at low levels of exposure to ionizing radiations, select the scientific basis it recommends the [federal agencies responsible for radiation protection] use, make such estimates of risk as it deems scientifically appropriate, [and] clearly delineate the interpretation and meaning that can be attributed to the estimates of risks when they are made," reviewing risks broadly and engaging the best scientific experts available for the task. The report provided guidelines by which both industrial and governmental agencies could set standards. The standards applying to the many devices which emit radiation—medical and dental X-ray machines, industrial and security X-ray devices, radioactive cobalt, radium, and iodine used in medicine, electronic devices such as television sets, and nuclear power plants—must be based on such overall assessments, as must standards for occupational exposure of those who mine radioactive minerals, make X-ray inspections of welded seams, or otherwise work around radiation.[43]

Such critical reviews serve to confirm data that are reliable and reveal those in need of further attention, and they often launch a subsequent round of investigation. The process is iterative; each cycle of inquiry improves upon the previous one. The need for flexibility and periodic reassessment has been emphasized by the Health, Education, and Welfare Secretary's Commission on Pesticides:

> In weighing potential health risks against potential benefits it must never be forgotten that even the most far-seeing view may be proved erroneous by unexpected new scientific developments or by an altered attribution of those risks considered to be utmost importance. An instance may be cited in the area of nonnutritive sweeteners. Earlier safety evaluations took into

---

[43]National Academy of Sciences/National Research Council, Advisory Committee on the Biological Effects of Ionizing Radiation, *The Effects on Populations of Exposure to Low Levels of Ionizing Radiation* (1972). For commentary on this report see Arthur B. Tamplin, "The BEIR Report: A Focus on Issues," *Bulletin of the Atomic Scientists/Science and Public Affairs,* 19-20 (March 1973); and "The BEIR Report," *ibid.,* 47-49 (March 1973).

account softening of stools as the likely risk presented by high intake of cyclamates. Now one source of concern is the possibility of carcinogenesis brought about by these products or materials derived from them. Thus safety evaluation is an edifice whose construction is never completed; nor does it remain functional without periodic reconstruction. Strangely enough, both regulatory agencies and the public view as loss of face the frank recognition that many earlier decisions on safety must inevitably be proved wrong as scientific knowledge grows. There is nothing absolute about such decisions. All that we have a right to expect at the time they are made is that they should be the products of scientific competence and experience, mature judgment and full possession of all existing data.[44]

ASSEMBLING THE EVIDENCE

Experimenting on Human Subjects

The uniqueness of the evolutionary path *Homo sapiens* has taken means that although experiments on other species are absolutely necessary, they cannot substitute for studying man himself.

Tests on humans are essential. This century's extraordinary pharmaceutical progress, for instance, would not have been possible without the experiments carried out on thousands of volunteer subjects. The same is true for a great diversity of pesticides, food preservatives, cosmetics, and therapeutic and nutritional agents.

Precedent was set early in the century by those concerned about the safety of food additives. As the nation became industrialized and an increasing proportion of its food was preserved and processed for movement in commerce, the new food industry found it advantageous to add chemicals to the food to preserve it and enhance its saleability. The history of that era makes fascinating reading and impresses one with how much the situation has improved.[45]

In 1911, the first important study of the safety of the artificial sweetener, saccharin, was made for the Department of Agriculture.

---

[44]U. S. Department of Health, Education, and Welfare, *Report of The Secretary's Commission on Pesticides and Their Relationship to Environmental Health* (1969).

[45]Ruth de Forest Lamb, *American Chamber of Horrors. The Truth about Food and Drugs* (Farrar & Rinehart, New York, 1936); Oscar E. Anderson, *The Health of a Nation: Harvey W. Wiley and the Fight for Pure Food* (University of Chicago Press, 1958); James Harvey Young, "The science and morals of metabolism: catsup and benzoate of soda," *Journal of the History of Medicine and Allied Sciences 23*, 86-104 (1968); James Harvey Young, *The Toadstool Millionaires: A Social History of Patent Medicines in America before Federal Regulation* (Princeton University Press, Princeton, N. J. (1972).

Harvard professors Christian A. Herter and Otto Folin gave a dozen medical students fairly large doses (up to 1.5 grams a day) of saccharin. Their report concluded that "considering the number of men involved, the length of the experiment, and the amounts of saccharin given, the negative character of the results obtained indicates that, so far as can be ascertained with methods at present available, saccharin in moderate doses is not injurious to the health of normal, sound adults." The experiments were crude by today's standards; but the difficulty of the problem becomes apparent when one remembers that the risks of saccharin are not known with certainty even today.[46]

Much of what we know about DDT and other pesticides comes from human studies, and the effects of tetraethyl lead have been assessed by monitoring the metabolism of volunteers after they have inhaled the chemical.[47] Pharmaceuticals are screened systematically on human subjects before being put on the market. Durable consumer goods such as toys, home appliances, and construction tools, whose hazards lie mostly in discrete accidents, are tested by their manufacturers, sometimes on the firms' own employees and their families. Toys are sent home to employees' children. Cosmetics in the development stage are passed out to the office force in return for a later report. Such testing is clearly to the manufacturers' advantage, and it often leads to improvement of the products. It is not required by law. As with all studies on human subjects, serious questions of ethics need to be raised, as do questions of effectiveness in protecting the consumer public.

Despite all that society stands to gain from such studies, many promising investigations cannot be undertaken because of restraints of either practicality or propriety. As to practicality, it may be difficult to locate and engage a sufficient number of subjects, especially if persons having a certain metabolic disorder or some other specific physical or psychological characteristic are required. Remuneration may be costly. There are problems in selecting subjects, obtaining their informed consent, and arranging continuing postexperiment medical examinations. If the problem under scrutiny is one of mutagenesis, teratogenesis, or other delayed or multigenerational effect, the human life span and generation

---

[46]U. S. Department of Agriculture, Referee Board of Scientific Experts, "Influence of Saccharin on the nutrition and health of man," *USDA report no. 94* (1911); James Harvey Young, "Saccharin: A bitter regulatory controversy," in Frank B. Evans and Harold T. Pinkett, editors, *Research in the Administration of Public Policy* (Howard University Press, Washington, D. C., 1975).

[47]See chapter 6; R. A. Kehoe, "The metabolism of lead in health and in disease" (The Harben Lectures, 1960), *Journal of the Royal Institute of Public Health and Hygiene 24*, 1-203 (1969).

period may be so long as to force reliance on nonhuman organisms. This is especially true for imminent hazards demanding immediate, even if tentative, appraisals.

Beyond these restraints of practicality, there are profound issues of propriety and justice. Experiments must be ethically sound, reasonable in the opinion of professional peers of the investigators, allowed under the law, and justifiably beneficial to the subjects or to society. The historical record reveals some shameful exploitation as well as much entirely laudable work; the nation is currently examining these difficult issues in many forums.

Different kinds of subjects are employed. Historically and to some extent presently, investigators have often performed tests on themselves; one thinks of the early work on vaccines and anesthetics. For the discoverer of a new thing, the question, "Would you expose yourself or your family to it?" will always be a guiding criterion. Because of the desirability of maintaining continuous medical surveillance of the subjects, studies often employ military personnel, prisoners, inmates of corrective institutions, or medical students. Often, therapeutic measures can be tested only on patients afflicted with an illness. Medical students are used frequently, because they are generally healthy, able to understand what is being done and to notice abnormal signs themselves, and available for close observation where they live and work. In quite another area, home appliances, toys, and industrial tools are sometimes, but by no means always, tested on representative intended users during a test-marketing period before being put on general sale.

As human subjects have come to be used more and more, and as society's values have changed, protecting the rights of subjects has become of greater concern. A standard precaution by the medical and other professions has been to endorse codes of ethics. These principles can be traced from the Oath of Hippocrates, through the writings of the eighteenth- and nineteenth-century physician-experimenters Thomas Percival and Claude Bernard, up to contemporary codes of professional practice. Reacting to the atrocities of torture, experimentation, and pseudo-experimentation revealed by the Nuremberg war trials, the War Crimes Tribunal set a precedent in 1947 by establishing a strong code governing human experimentation.[48] In 1948 the World Medical Association adopted a "Declaration of Geneva" and in 1964 a "Declaration of Helsinki,"

---

[48]"Permissible Medical Experiments," in U. S. Adjutant General's Department, *Trials of War Criminals Before Nuremberg Military Tribunals Under Control Council Law No. 10 (October 1946-April 1949)*, vol. 2, 181-183 (U. S. Government Printing Office, Washington, D. C., 1947).

both of which were endorsed by a number of national medical organizations. The American Medical Association and other professional societies have devised their own, similar codes of conduct.

Most of these codes are based on the following cluster of precepts:

- The experimenter should fully disclose the nature of the test to the subject.
- Prior *voluntary, informed* consent should be secured from the subject.
- The benefits to the subject or to society should be sufficiently great to justify the experiment.
- All investigations should be under the close supervision of fully certified professionals.
- Every reasonable precaution against mishap should be taken.
- Both the subject and the investigator should be free to stop the experiment at any time.

Because codes cannot enforce themselves, most granting agencies and research institutions have adopted mechanisms for overseeing experimentation carried out under their auspices. The Department of Health, Education and Welfare has set guidelines governing all research it supports; for example, institutions are required to have a committee to conduct initial and continuing review of projects with respect to protection of the rights of the subjects, expectation of benefit to the subject and to humanity, adequacy of the consent obtained, and general adherence to standard codes of practice.[49] These federal guidelines are currently being revised, and the overall problem of human experimentation is being reviewed by a National Commission for the Protection of Human Subjects of Biomedical and Behavioral Research.[50]

Questions arise that are both grave and subtle. With the use of drugs in a large teaching hospital, when does slight modification of an established therapeutic procedure—and then a little more modification in the interest of improvement—cease being standard and become experimental? What constitutes *free* consent: does a prisoner feel no coercion when

---

[49]U. S. Department of Health, Education, and Welfare, *The Institutional Guide to DHEW Policy on Protection of Human Subjects* (1971).

[50]The Commission's first report discussed fetal research: National Commission for the Protection of Human Subjects of Biomedical and Behavioral Research, "Research on the fetus," 40 *Federal Register,* 33530-33552 (August 8, 1975).

asked to take part in a pesticide toxicity experiment, perhaps in return for much needed payment or for promise of favorable consideration for parole? Is it fair for a medical professor to ask his students, whose careers he can influence, to submit to a series of drug tests? What constitutes *informed* consent for an inmate of a mental institution, a child, a senile person, or, for that matter, any technically untrained person? The normative tenor of these questions has led many institutions to include members of the legal and other professions and citizens from the community at large in their review committees.

One cautious way of proceeding is to take a carefully graduated, phased, or staged approach to testing. Only after animal tests have set some of the boundaries and indicated what organ systems are likely to be affected do human tests begin. At first, a few closely monitored subjects are employed. Then as sufficient understanding is acquired to ensure the safety of subjects in the next stage, more are involved. Eventually, if indications are favorable, large-scale trials are undertaken. Such an approach is routine in the testing of new pharmaceuticals, and it is usually recommended for the testing of food additives, pesticides, detergents, cosmetics, contraceptive devices, and other agents to which the public is widely exposed.

New questions are now being raised about studies on fetuses and aborted fetuses, the rights of prisoners and the mentally infirm, the management of pharmaceutical research, the conduct of behavioral experiments, and the supervision of non-federally-funded research.[51]

We have said that deliberate testing on humans is essential, but that there are severe limitations of both practicality and propriety. Great ethical questions are involved. To those who argue that these experiments should be prohibited, we must point out that unless commerce ceases altogether, prohibition of controlled testing would simply convert society at large into even more of an uncontrolled, gigantic test laboratory than it already is. Forsaking the testing of new products on closely observed

---

[51]National Academy of Sciences/National Research Council, *Use of Human Subjects in Safety Evaluation of Food Chemicals* (1967); "Ethical aspects of experimentation with human subjects," *Daedalus 98*, no. 2, 219-594 (Spring 1969); Irving Ladimer, editor, "New dimensions in legal and ethical concepts for human research," *Annals of the New York Academy of Sciences 169*, 293-593 (1970); U. S. Senate, Subcommittee on Health of the Committee on Labor and Public Welfare, *Hearings on Human Experimentation* (February 21-23 and March 6-8, 1973); Bernard Barber, John J. Lally, Julia Loughlin Makarushka, and Daniel Sullivan, *Research on Human Subjects. Problems of Social Control in Medical Experimentation* (Russell Sage Foundation, New York, 1973), reviewed by David Mechanic in *Science 181*, 255-256 (1973); Sissela Bok, "The ethics of giving placebos," *Scientific American 231*, 17-23 (November 1974); National Academy of Sciences, *Experimentation and Research with Humans: A Conflict in Value* (1975).

subjects would default those experiments onto unwary consumers, from whom the rest of us would probably never learn anything. Doing away with supervised testing of toys by their manufacturers would simply shift the experiments to the nation's playrooms.

Reviewing Inadvertent and Occupational Exposure

In Iraq in late 1971 the most serious epidemic of methylmercury poisoning ever recorded broke out. Wheat and barley had been imported for planting to help relieve a near famine. Following common practice in the Western nations from which they were imported, the seeds had been treated with antifungal preservative compounds of mercury. When the grain reached the rural areas, some desperate farm families diverted part of the seeds to their kitchens for making bread. Besides not being warned sufficiently, the Iraqis misunderstood the hazard: they thought that since the red warning dye could be washed off the seeds, that the poison was also eliminated. Some, not knowing that signs of mercury poisoning may not appear for days, took it as an indication of safety that chickens fed samples of the treated grain did not immediately show any adverse effects. By January of 1972 hundreds of people with the neural agonies of mercury poisoning were making their way to hospitals every day. Before the epidemic ended 6,530 cases of poisoning were admitted to hospitals and 459 deaths were recorded. In such a rural setting it is not unlikely that other cases went unreported.

No one would deliberately feed near-lethal or lethal doses of mercury compounds to human beings. However, when such ingestion occurred accidentally, it was imperative that the rest of the world learn as much as possible from the accident. In this case investigators from several nations rushed in to collaborate and glean whatever lessons might be available. Invaluable information was obtained about the metabolic route of mercury through the body, about how the poison is cleared from the body, and about the comparative efficacy of several medications. The symptoms of acute poisoning were described: loss of sensation in the hands and feet and around the mouth, loss of coordination in gait, slurring of speech, and eventually deafness, blindness, and death. Rough dose-effect relationships were estimated.[52]

---

[52]F. Bakir, S. F. Damluji, L. Amin-Zaki, M. Murtadha, A. Khalidi, N. Y. Al-Rawi, S. Tikriti, H. I. Dhahir, T. W. Clarkson, J. C. Smith, and R. A. Doherty, "Methylmercury Poisoning in Iraq," *Science 181*, 239-241 (1973).

The mercury compounds involved in this terrible epidemic are widely distributed items of commerce with many uses. There have been other instances of poisoning, both in manufacturing and in agricultural handling, and there have been several outbreaks of epidemic poisoning besides the one in Iraq. Terrible long-term mercury poisoning, "Minamata disease," was inflicted during 1953-1960 upon hundreds of Japanese who had eaten fish from waters tainted with mercuric waste from plastics industries.[53] In identifying the modes of hazard, in relating exposure to effect, in setting standards and controlling exposure, studying these accidents has given us information we could not have gained in any other way.

Even the tragedies of war have their lessons: much of what we know about the induction of leukemia and other illnesses by radiation comes from follow-up medical studies of the survivors of the Hiroshima and Nagasaki atomic bomb explosions. We learn from those having inborn deficiencies of metabolism and from those who are for some reason especially susceptible to certain hazards. For example, the reaction of especially sensitive people's skin to toiletries, cosmetics, detergents, and industrial materials has implications for the rest of the population; if sensitive people suffer obvious, quick reaction, others who are less sensitive may be undergoing less obvious but nonetheless undesirable reactions.

Extremely valuable information can be gained from occupational experience. Because exposure in the workplace is likely to be consistent and repeated, the conditions of exposure can be determined with some precision. Often, exposure has been endured for a long time. Even if the current hazard to the general public is slight, as might be the case for a new product, there are under the roof of the manufacturer a number of persons already exposed in the course of development and early manufacture. Workers have been said to serve in this sense as "miners' canaries" for the rest of the population.

There are substantial obstacles to following up on accidental and occupational exposure. Emergencies usually catch investigators unprepared; control groups may not exist; and, of course, therapy must take precedence over research. If investigators were better prepared to undertake them, emergency studies would be more effective. But to dispatch established scientists, fully equipped, off to Iraq on a moment's notice isn't easy.

---

[53]Philip H. Abelson, *Science 169*, 237 (1970); poignant pictorial documentation is presented in W. Eugene Smith and Aileen M. Smith, *Minamata* (Holt, Rinehart and Winston, New York, 1975).

The domestic accident studies conducted by the Consumer Product Safety Commission hold promise; the detective work that pins down why a television set burst into flame or electrocuted someone has implications not only for immediate remedial action but also for improving the product's basic design. The study of occupational hazards is frustrated by the defensive, but in principle understandable, reluctance of manufacturers to open their doors and files to outsiders. With researchers, unions, representatives of public interest groups, and the press clamoring for access to "the facts," and with the corporation management scrambling, hedging, and pressing its own researchers for irrefutable substantiation or disproof of what may at that point be only a suspicion, pursuing the matter in a careful, orderly fashion may be almost impossible.

Making Epidemiological Surveys

"Guilt by association"—the principle of the epidemiological method—clearly has its weaknesses. But it sometimes delivers a surprisingly strong indictment of hazards that have managed to evade other techniques, and it can supplement experimentation in several useful ways. Often epidemiological evidence provides an early warning which induces investigators to study a threat further by other methods; this has been one of the major effects of the epidemiological studies implicating smoking as a cause of cancer.[54]

Basically, the epidemiological approach compares several groups that are similar *except* with respect to some particular factor—exposure, genetic makeup, age, sex, or whatever. The questions take the form: "Do spraymen using this insecticide suffer more liver disease than farm workers having similar physiologies and social standing (with its implications of lifestyle, diet, medical care, and so on) but who are not exposed to the spray?" "Do children going to school near noisy jetports have a greater tendency to become schizophrenic than similar children living in quieter places?" "Do babies exposed to X-rays while in the womb show an increased tendency to develop birth defects?" "Do people drinking fluoridated water enjoy better dental health than those drinking water that is not fluoridated?"

The difficulties of selecting subjects, collecting data in the field, analyzing piles of statistical data, and reaching convincing conclusions are appreciable. One of the method's most serious shortcomings is its

---

[54] A good general text is John P. Fox, Carrie E. Hall, and Lila R. Elvaback, *Epidemiology and Disease* (MacMillan, N. Y., 1970).

ineffectiveness in proving that effect results from cause: the statistics do show that smokers suffer a higher incidence of throat cancer, but in what logical sense does that prove that smoking *causes* the cancer? (Does smoking simply aggravate incipient cancer? Are there other causes predisposing to both a preference for smoking and susceptibility to cancer?)

Experimenting on Nonhuman Organisms

Mice, rats, guinea pigs, rabbits, hamsters, dogs, cats, monkeys, cows, pigeons, pigs—along with others, these animals have served to tell us how much cadmium is lethal, which organs are most susceptible to damage from radiation, and whether certain drugs taken by expectant women will leave their babies unharmed. The use of lower animals as substitutes or models for human subjects is so familiar that the term "guinea pig" has become a colloquialism. For most people, any qualms over jeopardizing the animals are more than offset by the desire to gain knowledge useful in alleviating human suffering.

Experimenting with animals makes possible the use of very large numbers of subjects, thereby assuring more reliable data. One ambitious study was conducted by the Oak Ridge National Laboratory in an effort to assess the effects of very-low-level radiation like that released by medical devices and nuclear power plants. It was known that the effects, if any, would be quite subtle. So in the interest of making significant observations, thousands of genetically homogeneous mice were housed through their entire lives near weak radiation sources. Routine examinations and autopsies of the mice revealed important information, especially about the relation between the radiation dose and the incidence of cancer.[55] Such so-called (but misnamed) "mega-mouse experiments" have helped provide a base for setting radiation exposure standards. Other studies of radiation have followed the genetic and teratogenic health of mice through many generations—the kind of experiments this fast-moving age has no time to wait for with human subjects.

On animals, experiments can be performed that would be unacceptably hazardous to human subjects. Large control groups can be maintained, thus providing reliable bases for comparison. Groups of animals can be treated in different ways and not all kept identically healthy, a practice generally forbidden with human subjects for ethical reasons.

[55]Arthur C. Upton *et al.*, "Quantitative experimental study of low-level radiation carcinogenesis," *International Atomic Energy Agency Conference* no. IAEA-SM118/6, 425-438 (Vienna, 1969); John B. Storer, "The low level experiment," *Oak Ridge National Laboratory Review 5*, no. 4, 1-5 (1972).

Following the recognition that is is often desirable to minimize genetic dissimilarities among test subjects, large colonies of genetically homogeneous animals have been developed; inbred strains of many different kinds of animals are now available. These animal stocks have come to be considered a resource just as valuable as collections of rare chemicals or apparatus. However, using inbred animals may not always be advisable; there is often disagreement over whether inbred strains are preferable to less homogeneous ones. This problem has been described, with specific reference to mutagenicity testing but with implications for other research as well:

> It does not seem possible at present to determine quantitatively what fraction of the human population is at increased mutational risk because of genetically determined high mutagenic susceptibility, and this factor cannot therefore now be taken into account when computing average susceptibilities. The main significance of variable susceptibility lies in its implications for the choice of suitable organisms for screening programs. Most screening systems employ specially chosen (that is, highly inbred) strains, which may not be representative of natural populations. It is therefore desirable to obtain comparative individual data on mutagenic susceptibility, particularly for men ... As a general principle, mutagenicity screening should, where possible, be conducted using genetically diverse populations.[56]

Using inbred strains does simplify the system to be analyzed. But the process of breeding in certain characteristics of, say, coat color, may breed out less obvious characteristics—perhaps the susceptibility to the very hazard one is concerned about. Deep-seated metabolic sensitivities, which are hard to detect, may be lost. The inbred strain may then react deceptively more mildly than highly varying, less inbred animals (and the humans they are standing in for), leading to serious underestimation of the risk.

The day-to-day practical difficulties of managing animal experiments almost have to be endured personally to be appreciated: feeding uniformly and on schedule, keeping the cages, tanks, or stalls clean, controlling the ambient temperature, protecting the animals from disease and vermin, keeping records, collecting specimens, arranging matings, performing deliveries, shielding the young from harm, conducting autopsies, and in general taking every possible measure to ensure that whatever unusual

---

[56]Environmental Mutagen Society, committee 17, "Environmental mutagenic hazards," *Science 187*, 503-514 (1975).

effects are observed will not be due to uncontrolled or unnoticed variation in experimental conditions but will be solely and compellingly attributable to the hazard under suspicion. And this perhaps with many hundreds or thousands of smelly, squealing, squirming, defecating, biting animals. Few people would engage in such work were it not so essential.

Testing Product Performance

Many products are amenable to dynamic or performance testing. Reaction to stress is measured, either in normal or simulated use or under highly taxing, exaggerated conditions. A hair dryer is run for a long time to test its tendency to short-circuit and leak current to the outer casing. Window glass is flexed, scratched, and thumped to gauge its resistance to shattering. An automobile brake part is "worked" repeatedly until it fails. The principle is familiar: "If the limb can support Father's weight, it should be a safe one for a swing."

Standardizing the test conditions may be important. A manufacturer of window glass wants to be able to subject his panes to identical tests day after day, year after year. Industry-wide steel testing requires comparability. The Food and Drug Administration has to authorize standard bacterial food contamination tests for the entire nation.

The appropriateness of the tests is a second consideration. What standard conditions should be chosen? It is probably fair to say that most test methods "just grow" (which does not necessarily mean that the process is haphazard), and that pressures from industrial, government, military, and consumer groups strongly influence the evolution of standard tests. Often the conditions are chosen to simulate real use. Electrical applicances are tested at normal household voltages. Tires are tested under the loads they are expected to carry and under grueling road conditions, as the tire industry so dramatically demonstrates in its television advertisements. But since every product has as many properties as one might wish to measure, which ones should be looked at? The problem is illustrated by a difficulty encountered in setting flammability standards for fabrics used for children's bedclothing: in general, changing a fabric's composition to raise its ignition temperature—the point at which it bursts into flame—also raises its resistance to extinction once ignited; should bedclothing flammability tests and standards emphasize ease of ignition, or ease of extinction?

Dismayingly, Harvard engineer and combustion specialist Howard Emmons has said that "although the data on fires over the century are not very reliable, they do suggest that the success of fire-control measures is not significantly greater now than it was in earlier times.'' Flammability testing is part of the difficulty.

The problems in this area are suggested by the remarkable discrepancy from country to country in judgments on what is flammable. For example, in the early 1960's each of six nations undertook (in cooperation with the International Organization for Standardization) to rate 24 wall-covering materials in order of their flammability according to that nation's standard test. The results disagreed widely.

The serious nature of the disagreement between different ''standards'' was shown by material No. 18, a phenolic-foam wallboard; it was the safest of all 24 materials according to the standard test in Germany and the most hazardous of all 24 according to Denmark's test. On the other hand, material No. 7, an acrylic-sheet wallboard, was the third safest material by the Danish test and the third most flammable by the German. . . .

What the scatter of the test results means is that no one knows what characteristics a material should have to be safe in a fire. Each of the national tests was based on a best judgment rather than on rigorously established facts, and so each test measured something different under the heading of flammability. It was inevitable that the results would diverge.

The development of an improved approach requires that the basic nature of fire in a building be understood well enough to devise a test that measures the right characteristics. In fact, a little thought shows that the present approach of assigning a single value to indicate the flammability of a material is basically wrong. As every Boy Scout knows, one cannot make a campfire with a single log; it takes at least two and preferably more. A single log does not have an inherent fire-safety measure. Only the entire system involved in a potential fire can be rated.

Eventually building codes will have to be rewritten to rate rooms and buildings rather than single materials. I say eventually because at present not enough is known to provide a basis for rating a room. Before such a rating can be made the materials themselves will have to be subjected to a number of separate tests that measure the ease of ignition, the rate of spread of fire, the production of smoke and toxic gas and other characteristics, which can then be combined for a given room into a measure of its flammability and hence of its acceptability in a home or a public building.[57]

The degree to which the tests should anticipate product misuse is a third consideration. Should a meat grinder, a clothes wringer, or an industrial punch press be rated for ''proper'' use only, or should the straying of fatigued, youthful, or distracted hands also be anticipated?

---

[57]Howard W. Emmons, "Fire and fire protection," *Scientific American 231*, 21-27 (July, 1974).

An impressive repertoire of tests has been developed by such organizations as the American Society for Testing and Materials, Underwriters Laboratories, the engineering societies, the military, and the government agencies. With the adoption of these standard tests a manufacturer can order aluminum or glass or polyester fiber of a specified rating from a supplier and have full confidence in the performance properties of the material. For the ultimate consumer of the product this helps assure uniformity and dependability. Obviously, the fact that standards exist does not mean that things meet them, and the fact that things meet standards does not imply that the standards are high; those are matters of quality control and value judgment.

Destructive testing, in which a material is subjected to stress until it fails, is often useful. Wire cables used in construction are stretched or flexed repeatedly in a heavy testing machine until they break, providing a measure of their strength. Mattreses have a heavy weight bounced on them thousands of times until the springs fail. Glass bottles are subjected to increasing internal pressure until they explode.

For some products, actual *in-use testing* is desirable. So manufacturers run test kitchens, send prototypes home with employees for evaluation, and move products onto the market by using a test-marketing strategy in which the opinions of early users are solicited by follow-up surveys.

Because of the near impossibility of anticipating every circumstance of misuse, and because product variation and the limitations of assembly-line sampling prevent perfect review of products, a *safety factor* is often applied. The numbers are usually arbitrary. One sees such designations as "safety factor 30%" (meaning that the product has been tested without failure at stresses up to 30% greater than design "normal use" specifications) or "use at no more than 500 pounds per square inch; tested to 1200 pounds per square inch."

PROBLEMS OF INFERENCE

Relating effects to their causes. Deciding whether experimental findings are significant. Extrapolating from animals to man. Sorting out synergistic and antagonistic effects. Pinning down subtle low-level phenomena. These are some of the inferential problems that must be overcome in making the leap from experiments to conclusions.

Relating Cause with Effect

Unavoidably, proofs of causality are tenuous. Findings are always open to new interpretation as additional experiments are completed or as other knowledge becomes available. The problem is greater with long-range, delayed effects.

In 1964 the committee charged with advising the Surgeon General on whether smoking causes cancer had to evaluate piles of conflicting reports. Controversy was inevitable. Nevertheless, the panel had to draw whatever conclusions the existing knowledge supported. Anticipating the questions that were bound to come, the committee outlined its criteria of causality:[58]

> Statistical methods cannot establish proof of a causal relationship in an association. The causal significance of an association is a matter of judgment which goes beyond any statement of statistical probability. To judge or evaluate the causal significance of the association between the attribute or agent and the disease, or effect upon health, a number of criteria must be utilized, no one of which is an all-sufficient basis for judgment. These criteria include:
>
> a) The consistency of the association
> b) The strength of the association
> c) The specificity of the association
> d) The temporal relationship of the association
> e) The coherence of the association.

That study's conclusion—that smoking does increase a person's chances of developing cancer—is familiar. But, ten years and several revisions later, the strength of the causal proof is still debated. The committee admitted to agonizing: "Various meanings and conceptions of the term *cause* were discussed vigorously at a number of meetings of the committee and its subcommittees. These debates took place usually after data and reports had been studied and evaluated; and at the time when critical scrutiny was being given to conclusions and to the wording of conclusive statements."[59]

In another instance, the problem was to determine whether radioactive dusts and gases were causing lung cancer among uranium miners. Was the disease solely due to the radioactivity, or was dust inhalation an aggravating factor? More than thirty-four hundred uranium miners and millers working in the Colorado Plateau area were studied epidemiologically; attempts were

---

[58]U. S. Surgeon General's Advisory Committee on Smoking and Health, *Smoking and Health,* 20 (1964).

[59]Also see Stanley Joel Reiser, "Smoking and health: The Congress and causality," 293-311 of Sanford A. Lakoff, editor, *Knowledge and Power* (The Free Press, New York, 1966).

made to correct for such "confounding variables" as differences in recentness of exposure and in the men's history of cigarette smoking. The report listed its causal criteria:[60]

> To evaluate the causal significance of airborne radiation in respiratory cancer, several criteria will be utilized, no one of which is definitive by itself. These criteria are as follows:
>
> the demonstration of an excess risk
>
> the demonstration of a dose-response relation
>
> the persistence of the excess risk and the dose-response relation
>
> the consistency of the association
>
> the specificity of the association
>
> the distinctive distribution of respiratory cancers according to anatomic site and histologic type.

The study found a higher mortality among the uranium miners than among other comparable males in that area, and it attributed the lung cancer to inhalation of the radioactive dusts and gases in the mines. Tying its findings to other evidence, the report cited experiments in which laboratory animals exposed to inhaled insoluble radioactive particles developed lung cancer, and it reviewed other epidemiological studies showing that "an excess in mortality from lung cancer has not ordinarily been shown without substantial exposure to radioactive materials." It also cited as being consistent a report that fluorospar miners exposed to radioactive gases develop respiratory cancer with an unusually high frequency. These pieces of evidence together were taken as proof that the radioactivity of the inhaled dust and gases of the uranium mines causes lung cancer in the miners.

Although they deal with two different hazards and are expressed in different language, the above sets of criteria are similar. These same criteria govern our everyday reasoning as well: a phenomenon is thought to be *caused* by something else if the two are found strongly in association and one in some essential sense precedes the other; if diminishing the presumed causal factor results in a lessening of the effect; if the observation is specific; if the occurrence in association persists; and so on.

---

[60]Joseph K. Wagoner, Victor E. Archer, Frank E. Lundin, Jr., Duncan A. Holaday, and J. William Lloyd, "Radiation as the cause of lung cancer among uranium miners," New England Journal of Medicine 273, 185 (1965); see also Frank E. Lundin, Jr., Joseph K. Wagoner, and Victor E. Archer, Radon Daughter Exposure and Respiratory Cancer. Quantitative and Temporal Aspects (U. S. Department of Health, Education, and Welfare, NIOSH/NIEHS joint monograph no. 1 (1971).

Much of safety investigation is detective work. One important technique is *accident-chain analysis*. Events leading to harm are analyzed in an attempt to reconstruct their sequence of occurrence, with a precipitating event causing a subsequent event causing another event, and so on to the final damage. (Mrs. O'Leary's cow kicked over the lantern, which ignited the hay, which fired the barn, which eventually sent the whole Windy City up in smoke. . . .)

An elderly woman, wearing her lacy houserobe as she cooks breakfast, reaches over a lighted front burner on her gas range to adjust a knob on the stove's back panel; the burner ignites her frilly cuff, and she is badly burned before she can extinguish the flames.[61] This is the sort of case that can be examined by accident-chain analysis, with the purpose of determining causal relations and looking for a way to break the chain and thus prevent the accident. In this case, educating the users, flameproofing the fabric, redesigning the garment, and changing the placement of knobs on the stove have been recommended as preventive measures. Analysis of many similar accidents has revealed contributory circumstances which can be seen as a syndrome: "Clothing ignition resulting when the victim reached across a stove primarily involved young girls and elderly women . . . nearly three-fifths of the cases occurred during the morning hours . . . in nearly one-half of the cases involving victims beyond age 65, robes and housecoats were the first fabric to ignite . . ."

Variations of this approach are used to investigate household, automobile traffic, and industrial accidents; similar but more elaborate techniques ("fault tree analysis") have been used to analyze hypothetical nuclear reactor accidents.[62]

In general one can distinguish several sorts of causal factors. The event at Mrs. O'Leary's is not at all a bad example: there were *predisposing* circumstances, with all the ingredients for a conflagration gathered in one place; there were precipitating, or *initiating,* actions, by the cow and maybe by Mrs. O'. herself; and there were contributory, *sustaining* causes that turned a minor accident into a disaster.

---

[61]This is a composite case which forms the cover illustration and pages 61-69 of the Secretary of Health, Education, and Welfare's *Flammable Fabrics,* fourth annual report to the President and the Congress, 1972.

[62]U. S. Atomic Energy Commission, *An assessment of accident risks in U. S. commercial nuclear power plants,* AEC WASH-1400 (August, 1974); for a critique of the AEC report's use of fault tree analysis, see Sierra Club/Union of Concerned Scientists, Henry W. Kendall and Sidney Moglewer, preparors, *Preliminary Review of the AEC Reactor Safety Study* (November, 1974).

Is the Difference Significant?

Determining risk is a business of making comparisons. Tests are run; a difference is observed. Is the difference simply a chance happening? Or is the difference *significant,* to be taken as a sign of truly different effect?

This kind of question brings into play some profound, fundamental notions. One of these is deeply rooted in everyday experience: if we want to know about a large group of events or objects, we examine a sample *(in judging a basket of peaches, we look at the peaches on top)*. A sample of only a few objects may leave us uneasy, so we enlarge the sample *(we check a few more peaches, perhaps from lower down)*. We continue to enlarge our sample until we are convinced that we have gained a significant view of the whole—or, put another way, that the difference between the average sample quality and the average quality of the entire group of objects is slight.

In a complex process not usually thought about explicitly, we have made a remarkably complicated decision that takes many factors into account. In general, the larger the lot, the larger the sample we examine *(we would check more peaches before buying a truckload than we would before buying a bushel)*. The greater the lot's variability, the more we worry whether we have sampled enough *(we would check more peaches if the assortment were varied than if the lot seemed to be uniform)*. We appreciate the need to sample in an unbiased way *(squeezing peaches from the bottom of the pile as well as the top)*.

Sampling is obviously essential when one can't examine every single item in a lot because of limitations of time or expense or access, or when testing damages the items. Proper sampling is critical in monitoring the environment, controlling product quality, and gathering epidemiological and experimental evidence in general. The intuitive notions outlined above are amenable to mathematical analysis, and some well developed mathematical techniques are available for application to practical problems.[63]

Because it is so essential to experimentation, and because it lies at the heart of so many regulatory controversies, the problem of deciding how important experimentally observed differences are deserves a bit more discussion. This problem arises in the form: "How many experiments are 'enough'?" "How many rabbits should this cosmetic ingredient be tested

---

[63]W. G. Cochran, *Sampling Techniques,* second edition (Wiley, New York, 1963); Ronald A. Fisher, *Statistical Methods and Scientific Inference,* revised edition (Hafner Publishing Company, New York, 1973).

on—ten, a hundred, a thousand?" Or in the interpretive stage, "The treated group's responses differed from the untreated group's by only a percent or so; would we be justified in concluding that the difference in treatment caused the difference in response?" The aim is to decide whether an observed difference should be attributed to the causal factor in question, or whether it might simply have occurred spontaneously, "by chance." Or, in cases in which no difference is observed, the question is whether any conclusion at all is warranted, and if so, what confidence we should place in it. For guidance we turn to statistical analysis.

[Before we take this brief overview any further we must state forcefully, but by no means derogatorily, that statistics cannot decide for us what is truth and what is not. After all, these frail numbers tenuously imposed on the situation are ours, not Nature's. Surprisingly often, we do get away with reasoning inductively, but even the best minds are hard pressed to explain how. Statistical analysis deserves to be appreciated as a powerful adjunct to, and an integral part of, experiment and observation. But as with any tool its usefulness will be enhanced if its inherent limitations are properly recognized. Now to see what it *can* do.]

Statistical analysis is commonly called upon to appraise tests for what might be called their inferential adequacy: the adequacy of a sample to represent the whole from which it was selected, the sensitivity of a test to pick up the difference between natural disease incidence and additional disease induced by different treatment. By inferential adequacy we mean the power of the tests to support or rule out conclusions. *"Checking just those five lovely peaches on top isn't an adequate test of the whole bushel."* Or, *"Because of the way peach trees vary, our simple experiment of spraying one of the two neighboring trees will not be very conclusive, no matter what its results."* Inferential adequacy is a performance characteristic of the test designs themselves.

In specific cases, given the numbers and adopting certain assumptions about the way things vary, we can appraise the power of the tests. As is intuitively clear from the peach-testing analogy, we have to consider the size of the overall lot (the "population"), the size of the experimental samples, the variation of the population and the samples, and the natural incidence and experimental occurrence of the effects in question. For present purposes we need not understand how the answers are actually calculated, but we should understand what they imply.

Suppose that two similar groups of 100 test animals are compared. One group is exposed to a suspected carcinogen, while the other is kept unexposed as a control group. Suppose then that no animals in either group develop cancer. Does this allow us to conclude that the agent never causes cancer? Clearly not. We ask how adequate the test is for examining the hypothesis that the agent causes cancer. Statistical analysis offers guidance. Answering in the only terms available to it, analysis affirms, for example, that if the agent actually induces no more than 3.0 tumors per 100 animals, the test has a 5% chance of failing to detect any tumors (this is referred to as the 95% confidence level). Similarly, the test has a 1% chance of finding no tumors even though as many as 4.5 of the population of 100 really are afflicted (99% confidence level); and so on.

We intuitively expect that doing the same experiment on more animals would be better. It is. Using 1000 animals and finding no tumors, there is a 1% chance of missing up to 4.6 tumored animals out of 1000 (or 0.46 per 100, as compared to 4.6 per 100 for the test using tenfold fewer animals). The more subjects, the better the probe.

Time for a chart. Let us consider the test described above—one of the simplest cases—in which *no* tumors are detected in either the exposed subjects or the controls. We examine the tests fairly demandingly, expecting them to fail us no more than 1% of the time. Figure 2-11 depicts the highest tumor incidence that might pass undetected for given numbers of tests.

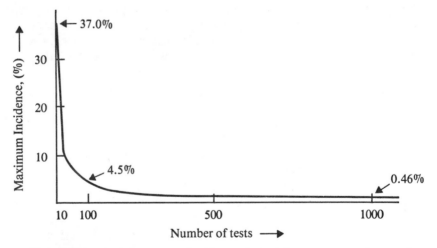

Figure 2-11. Maximum tumor incidence that might pass tests undetected (at 99% confidence level), for increasing number of tests.*

*Adapted from N. Mantel and W. R. Bryan, " 'Safety' testing of carcinogenic agents," *Journal of the National Cancer Institute 27,* 455-470 (1961).

Thus, locating the points of a few paragraphs ago, we see that at the 99% confidence level, tests on 10 animals might fail to detect tumors actually affecting up to 37% of the population; tests on 100 animals might find no tumors even though as much as 4.5% of the population is actually tumored; and tests on 1000 animals might reveal no tumors even though 0.46% of the whole population, or about 5 animals, are afflicted. Viewing it another way, if the tumors do occur to more than 5 animals per 1000, a test on 1000 animals can be expected to reveal the effect—at the 99% confidence level. Similar curves can be constructed for other confidence levels.

Obviously this is all simply a matter of degrees of certainty. In estimating risk, the best we can do is determine, at given levels of confidence, the maximum effects that could pass particular experiments undetected. However, the significance analyses do provide guidance, especially for comparing different experiments, and they indicate how the informational return diminishes as more and more tests are run. The numbers provide perspective on the experiments.

One implication of these notions is exemplified by the following discomforting comment from a panel reviewing carcinogenicity tests for food additives and pesticides:

> Even with as many as 1000 test animals and using only 90% confidence limits, the upper limit yielded by a negative experiment [one revealing no tumors] is 2.3 cancers per 1000 test animals. No one would wish to introduce an agent into a human population for which no more could be said than that it would probably produce no more than two tumors per 1000. To reduce the upper limit of risk to two tumors per one million [at confidence limit of 99.9%] would require a negative result in somewhat more than three million test animals."[64]

Tenuous assumptions must be adopted in making the statistical analyses. Real test situations are usually much more complicated than the simple hypothetical cases we used for illustration above. For instance, when the effect being assayed, such as cancer or mutation, occurs as a background or natural incidence, analysis is far from simple. These numbers are only guides and may be little solace to a researcher or administrator agonizing over whether a food additive is stealthily killing people or whether microwaves, the basis of multi-million-dollar industries, are harming

---

[64]Food and Drug Administration Advisory Committee on Protocols for Safety Evaluation, "Panel on carcinogenesis report on cancer testing in the safety evaluation of food additives and pesticides," *Toxicology and Applied Pharmacology 20,* 431 (1971).

human beings. We are limited to appraising the inferential adequacy of our tests, hoping to gain some guidance on their importance for our conclusions.

Extrapolating from Animals to Man

From that point early in life when we are told that because carrots are good for rabbits' eyes they are good for ours, we learn to deal with the notion of extrapolating knowledge from animals to human beings. We also rather quickly learn to question such extrapolations.

Man is unique. Therefore any extrapolative step can only be a hesitant one. No animal is a best model for man; for any given experiment, one can only use the species that appears to be most like man in the aspects at question. For instance, to test the skin-sensitizing property of a cosmetic, one might apply the substance to the shaved skin of an animal with sensitive, human-like skin, such as the albino rabbit.

Adverse reaction in animals does not prove adverse effect in man, and lack of reaction in animals does not prove that man will not be affected. Even closely related species can differ widely in their responses. The literature is replete with "anomalous" reactions. For example, the median lethal dose (LD_{50}) for the physiologically active compound histamine is 400 milligrams of histamine per kilogram body weight for rats and 200 milligrams per kilogram for mice, but less than 1 milligram per kilogram for rabbits and guinea pigs.[65] The infamous thalidomide, so horribly teratogenic to the human fetus, also causes birth defects in monkeys and rabbits— but not at all in rats.[66] In an extreme case, common table salt is, in massive amounts, teratogenic to mice: when injected under the skin (at 2500 milligrams salt per kilogram animal weight) of eleven-days-pregnant mice, it caused many of the offspring to have malformed digits, feet, and wrist and ankle joints.[67]

Clearly, drawing implications from any such tests requires care. (There is absolutely no evidence that salt at low doses causes human birth defects.) Yet for many purposes the tests are essential, as in the early phases of testing of new pharmaceuticals. Importantly, one retrospective

---

[65]C. A. Papcostas, E. R. Loew, and G. B. West, "Studies on the toxicology of a histamine liberator, compound 48-80," *Archives Internationales de Pharmacodynamie et de Thérapie 120,* 353 (1959).

[66]James G. Wilson, "Use of rhesus monkeys in teratological studies," *Federation* [of American Societies for Experimental Biology] *Proceedings 30,* 104-109 (1971).

[67]H. Nishimura and S. Miyamoto, "Teratogenic effects of sodium chloride in mice," *Acta Anatomica 74,* 121 (1969).

study of the toxicities of anticancer drugs with dogs and monkeys has confirmed that large-animal screenings over the long run have "served to alert the physician to a significant proportion of the total spectrum of drug effects, which were encountered during the clinical use of a new anticancer compound." That is, the animal tests proved to be valid predictors of later clinical experience.[68]

Several principles guide the planning and interpretation of such tests. Adverse reactions are respected, at least as warnings; if a cosmetic preparation rubbed onto a rabbit's skin causes a rash or blisters, this must be taken as a strong call for extensive skin sensitization testing. Second, although lower animals, being less expensive and easier to handle, are useful for preliminary screenings, they must be succeeded as subjects by higher mammals before a material is approved for human use.

A number of questions arise in designing the experiments.

What species should be used? The answer will be guided not only by economic considerations but also by experience with the physiology of the organ systems likely to be affected. For instance, chemicals suspected of neural toxicity must be screened on animals whose nervous system is as much like man's as possible.

How many tests should be run? This will be determined by the practical considerations of cost and feasibility, and by the degree of certainty desired.

What should be the mode of exposure in the test? For some hazards, such as noise, there is no question. But for others, such as asbestos—to which practical exposure may be respiratory (for asbestos workers), cutaneous (for users of talcum powder containing asbestos as an impurity), or ingestive (for people drinking a beverage filtered through asbestos) in different situations—choosing the test exposure may be more difficult. Even the details of administration can be important: one may find different results from administering a food additive by stomach tube rather than by simply feeding in a meal, or from giving a drug by intravenous injection, by injection into the skin, and by implanting the drug as a pellet under the skin.

---

[68]P. S. Schein, R. D. Davis, S. Carter, J. Newman, D. R. Schein, and D. P. Rall, "The evaluation of anti-cancer drugs in dogs and monkeys for the prediction of qualitative toxicities in man," *Clinical Pharmacology and Therapeutics 11*, 3-40 (1970).

How large should the dose be? Often the test exposure should simply be equivalent to, and in the form of, the exposure expected in everyday use. Complications arise when the effects are very weak, extremely rare, or delayed in onset; in those cases the only way to detect any response in the subjects may be to administer a dose many times that normally encountered. Such a procedure is always open to criticism, and extreme caution in drawing conclusions is warranted. At times, however, there may be no other way to obtain clues about the hazard.

How are dosages to be extrapolated from animals to man? Like many of the activities described in the preceding pages, extrapolation is almost an art. But some guidelines have been established. Practice has shown that for chemical substances the measure "milligrams of compound per kilogram of animal body weight," and more recently the measure "milligrams of compound per square meters of body area," can often be transferred directly in making comparisons between animals and man. In general, a compound having a certain physiological activity at some specified number of milligrams per square meter (or per kilogram) in test animals is *likely* at that level to have comparable activity in man, although there are so many anomalous cases that such extrapolations must always be viewed with skepticism.[69]

The above matters are pragmatic ones to which the only guide is experience. What works, works. One does, or reviews, the experiments, draws extrapolations as skillfully as possible in the light of experience, and cautiously proceeds to market the food additive, regulate the distribution of the industrial chemical, or conduct further tests of the drug. If no adverse repercussion ensues, one tentatively assumes that the extrapolation was valid. If, on the other hand, adverse findings begin to turn up in the scientific literature, or allergists begin making complaints, or legal suits are filed against the product, the extrapolation obviously has to be re-examined.

It is easy to appreciate that there might be disagreement about these judgments, especially in legal and regulatory decisions. Thus we find the Assistant Secretary of Labor for Occupational Safety and Health, in establishing regulations for the handling of certain industrial chemicals, having to say:

A major question of occupational carcinogensis relates to the extrapolation of results of animal experimentation to humans. The basis of numerous

---

[69]Emil J. Freireich, "Quantitative comparison of toxicity of anticancer agents in mouse, rat, hamster, dog, monkey, and man," *Cancer Chemotherapy Reports 50*, 219-244 (1966).

objections to the regulatory proposals is that, even assuming the validity of animal experiments, such do not furnish sufficient evidence that the substances involved are carcinogenic to humans. Extrapolation of results obtained by animal experimentation is alleged to be vitiated by several considerations: (a) that certain cancers are specific only to some species; (b) that the conditions of animal experiments are out of proportion to, and not consistent with, conditions prevailing in industrial exposure; and (c) that no cancers have yet been detected in humans exposed to the substances.

But he goes on to affirm, in the context of his rule-making responsibility, that "for those substances whose metabolism is understood, and is similar in both animals and man, the fact that they induce cancers in animals warrants the expectation that they will induce cancers in men."[70]

A general *caveat* was issued by the Food and Drug Administration's Panel on Carcinogenesis:

> Clearly extrapolation from the observable range to a safe dose has many of the perplexities and imponderables of extrapolation from animal to man, and it would be imprudent to place excessive reliance on mathematical sleight of hand, particularly when the dose-response curves used are largely empirical descriptions, lacking any theoretical physical or chemical basis.[71]

More research is urgently needed. Genetically homogeneous test animals must be compared to more heterogeneous, randomly bred ones whose sensitivities to hazards are more variable. Retrospective studies of the usefulness of various animals as predictors of human reactions are needed. And more attention must be given to the fundamental problems of controls, sampling, and other aspects of general experimental design.[72]

Sorting out Synergistic and Antagonistic Effects

Sulfur oxides are known to be bad for our lungs. So are smoke, soot, and other particulates. These major ingredients of air pollution apparently interact, in some way not fully understood, to affect health in a manner

---

[70]U. S. Department of Labor, Occupational Safety and Health Administration, "Occupational health and safety standards: Carcinogens," *39 Federal Register,* 3757 (January 29, 1974).

[71]Food and Drug Administration Panel on Carcinogenesis, "Panel on Carcinogenesis report on cancer testing in the safety evaluation of food additives and pesticides," *Toxicology and Applied Pharmacology 20,* 433 (1971).

[72]Leon Goldberg, editor, *Carcinogenesis Testing of Chemicals* (CRC Press, Cleveland, Ohio, 1974); National Academy of Sciences/National Research Council, *Principles for Evaluating Chemicals in the Environment* (1975).

different from that of any of the pollutants acting alone or simply additively.[73] We don't understand the effect of any single air pollutant very well, much less that of the complex mixtures constituting smog. If sulfur oxides and smoke enhance each other's adverse action on the lungs, what are the additional effects of carbon monoxide, nitrogen oxides, ozone, and peroxides, all of which, along with bacteria, dusts, viruses, and pollen, are commonly present in our metropolitan atmospheres?

There is a lot of speculation about agents acting in *synergistic* (reforcing, but more than simply additive) or *antagonistic* (opposing or neutralizing) manners, but we understand very little as yet. There is no doubt that such effects occur. Two modes of synergistic (and antagonistic) action can be distinguished: agents can interact in the environment to modify each other physically before affecting man; or the agents can mutually influence the body's reaction to each other. A creditable beginning has been made in understanding synergistic and antagonistic effects of medicinals and of some environmental pollutants, but we have far to go before we will understand the complex interactions of the mixtures to which we are exposed every day.

Evaluating Chronic, Low-level Agents

Conceptual, experimental, economic, legal, and regulatory distinctions can usefully be made between *acute, imminent hazards* and *chronic, low-level hazards*. Acute hazards are such things as kitchen knives, lye, and electrocuting currents. Chronic, low-level hazards include air pollutants, weak radiation, and asbestos dust. Notice that the terms *acute* and *low-level* refer to immediacy and intensity of action, not to seriousness of risk: a knife, an acute hazard, may cause only a minor cut, whereas a low-level carcinogen may prove deadly years after exposure. Here we will summarize the special problems of evaluating low-level hazards.

First, *the latent period may be very long*. (This is the period between exposure to a hazard and the onset of its effect). The latent period of some compounds known to cause cancer is shown in Table 2-3. Any studies of the effects of such slowly expressed agents will have to take this latency into account. And by obvious implication, short-range tests of new agents similar to these chemicals and radiation sources can only be regarded as tentative, pending the completion of protracted observations.[74]

---

[73]U. S. Department of Health, Education, and Welfare, *Air Quality Criteria for Sulfur Oxides,* 105-112 (1970).

[74]W. C. Heuper, "Environmental cancer," in F. Homburger and W. H. Fishman, editors, *Physiopathology of Cancer* (Albert J. Phiebig, White Plains, New York, 1959).

Table 2-3.   Latent period of some known carcinogens, for man.[74]

Carcinogen	Site of Cancer	Range of Latency (years)
X-rays	Skin	10-30
Radioactive paints	Bone	10-30
Radioactive ores	Lung	5-20
Ultraviolet exposure	Skin	10-40
Aromatic amines	Bladder	2-20
Coal tar (shale oil)	Skin	10-25
Soot (chimney sweeps)	Scrotum	11-17

Second, *a very large number of tests may be required for significance.* If deleterious effects occur with only low incidence, if the latent period is long, or if those adverse effects can also be due to other causes so that there is a background incidence (perhaps increasing with age), a very large number of observations may be required in order to demonstrate that the suspect agent does cause the damage.

Third, *very large doses may have to be administered in order to observe any effect.* This point has been debated heatedly in both the lay and scientific presses. It was central in the 1969 controversy over cyclamates, where it was expressed in the question, "Is the banning of cyclamate sweeteners warranted by the fact that they cause cancer in a few rats given extremely high doses for their entire lifetimes?"[75] The Food and Drug Administration later stated that "a 12 oz. bottle of soft-drink may have contained from ¼ to 1 gram of sodium cyclamate. An adult would have had to drink from 138 to 552 12 oz. bottles of soft-drink a day to get an amount comparable to that causing cancer in mice and rats."[76] In some cases the argument for such massive-dose experiments is simply that they are all that can be done. They do reveal clues as to the principal modes of action (showing, for instance, whether risk is principally to the liver, to the bladder, or to developing fetuses); this admittedly crude evidence can than be bolstered by evidence from other sources.

---

[75]Unsigned editorial, "How McPherson's Rule sank cyclamates," *Nature 224,* 398-399 (1969); see also Samuel S. Epstein, Alexander Hollaender, Joshua Lederberg, Marvin Legator, Howard Richardson, and Arthur H. Wolff, "Wisdom of cyclamate ban," *Science 166,* 1575 (1969).

[76]Letter from the Acting Commissioner of the Food and Drug Administration to the U. S. House of Representatives Committee on Appropriations, May 17, 1973, reprinted in *House Report on the Agriculture-Environmental and Consumer Protection Appropriation Bill, 1974,* Report No. 93-275 (1973).

One can certainly sympathize with public regulators who must make decisions about issues fraught with the above complications. In 1972 William Ruckelshaus, the administrator of the Environmental Protection Agency, footnoted these problems when he announced his agency's ban on DDT:

> It is particularly difficult to anticipate the long-range effects of exposure to a low dose of a chemical. It may take many years before adverse effects would take place. Diseases like cancer have an extended latency period. Mutagenic effects will be apparent only in future generations. Lastly, it may be impossible to relate observed pathology in man to a particular chemical because of the inability to isolate control groups which are not exposed in the same degree as the rest of the population.[77]

EXPRESSING RISK

All the complicated detective work we have been reviewing converges to meet the single purpose of estimating the probabilistic measure, *risk*. This is the output of the scientific effort; this becomes the input to personal and social decision making. Risk can be expressed in several ways.

Most expressions of risk are compound measures describing both the *probability* of harm and its *severity*. They may describe the risk to individuals, to particular groups, or to society as a whole. They are usually broad statistical measures that take into account the chance of being exposed as well as the chance of adverse effect from that exposure.

Thus in a familiar example, it is said that in the present year Americans on the average run a risk of about one in 4000 of dying in an automobile accident. The *probability* is one out of 4000 for injuries lethally *severe*. This projection is derived simply by noting that in the last few years there have been about 56,000 automobile deaths per year in a population of 224,000,000; this makes the risk to individuals on the average 56,000/224,000,000 or one in 4000 per year.[78] This expresses the overall risk to society; the risk to any particular individual obviously depends on his exposure, how much he is on the road, where he drives and in what weather, whether he is psychologically accident prone, what mechanical condition his vehicle is in, and so on.

Risks often need to be expressed in relation to exposure, so that different risks can be compared. In looking at the risks of different modes

---

[77] U. S. Environmental Protection Agency, "Consolidated DDT hearings," 37 *Federal Register,* 13369-13375, footnote 19 (July 7, 1972).

[78] National Safety Council, *Accident Facts* (1974).

of transportation, for instance, one might make comparisons in terms of mishaps per passenger mile: thus in 1972 the death rates per hundred million passenger miles were: for motorcycles, 17.0 deaths; for automobiles, 4.5 deaths (including nonpassengers); for commercial airplanes, 0.13 deaths.[79] One might similarly compare the number of disabling injuries per passenger hour, or death per rural mile or urban mile.

The Consumer Product Safety Commission has developed a product "risk index" as an aid to establishing its regulatory priorities. Devising the index has not been a simple task, and it is not yet finished. The version in use at this writing is a "Frequency-Severity Index," defined as the product of the frequency of injury and the severity. The frequency of injury is estimated from the National Electronic Injury Surveillance System (NEISS) analyses of hospital emergency room admissions.[80] The severity of injury is ranked on a scale assigning low numbers to such injuries as skin irritation and the highest to deaths. This index has helped the agency to establish priorities as it has begun its task of reducing the number of deaths and injuries from the more than 10,000 consumer products under its jurisdiction. The agency has struggled with the difficult problems of making the surveillance system workable and establishing the severity ratings in a reasonable way. Refinements have been made, and others are being considered. The index can now be adjusted for age of victims, in order to give extra weight to children's injuries. The commission is working on the problem of adjusting the index for extent of social hazard; a product rarely encountered should not be viewed as posing the same national threat as one having the same frequency and severity of injury, but which is in widespread use. Taking into account the number of the products sold or the number of hours they are used or the number used per day seems desirable, but that is very difficult and has not yet been done satisfactorily.[81]

The relatively straightforward figures we have been describing are commonly used to describe the risks of injury, illness, and death incurred from durable goods such as tools, home appliances, toys, and architectural hardware, and from accidents in transportation and manufacturing. The mortality figures can be converted into figures of life expectancy (average length of life). Risk indices can be devised. But for chronic hazards—ones that do not exert their effects immediately—expressing the risks is not so straightforward.

---

[79]National Safety Council, *Accident Facts* (1974).

[80]See p. 151ff.

[81]Steven Kelman, "Regulation by the numbers—a report on the Consumer Product Safety Commission," *The Public Interest 36,* 83-102 (1974).

One expression used for risks due to chronic hazards is simply the number of deaths due to the hazard. A recent report stated, "It is suggested that automobile emissions may account for as much as one quarter of one percent of the total urban health hazard. For the whole U.S. urban population, effects of this magnitude might represent as many as 4,000 deaths and 4 million illness-restricted days per year."[82] Another report has said that continued exposure of the American population to current levels of natural and manmade radiation causes 3,000 to 4,000 cancer deaths per year. Reading the details in that report reveals that the committee preparing it encountered serious difficulty in arriving at that estimate in the first place; that it had to make many assumptions (which the report documents); and that it acknowledges that other estimates besides the one it finally arrived at are plausible. The difficulty in using this risk expression is evidenced in the review and letters subsequently appearing in *Science* magazine.[83]

For some purposes, especially in elaborate, formal risk-benefit calculations, the expression, "extra deaths," has been used. In general, this expresses a change over time in the number of deaths due to specific causes. Its computation and interpretation can be highly controversial. One study estimated that among American men of all ages, there were about 11,000 "extra deaths" due to lung cancer in 1967, over the number there would have been in that year *if* the proportionate 1960 lung cancer death rate had obtained. "It is felt that these changes in death rates over a short period of years represent environmental changes in a broad sense ... the causes identified as contributing to the increase are ... [closely] related to ... environmental factors. ..."[84]

A somewhat similar description was used by the President's Science Advisory Committee in its 1972 report, *Chemicals and Health.* That report described societal risks in terms of "number who might be alive [if some exposure had been avoided]." Again the expression gauges broad trends. Again, its use is by no means simple, but as its PSAC expositors pointed out, "We would be more concerned about the difficulties of giving a

---

[82]National Academy of Sciences/National Research Council/National Academy of Engineering, *Air Quality and Automobile Emission Control,* prepared for the U. S. Senate Committee on Public Works, vol. 1, 13 (September, 1974).

[83]National Academy of Sciences/National Research Council, *The Effects on Populations of Exposure to Low Levels of Ionizing Radiation,* 364 (1972); *Science 178,* 966 (1972); *ibid. 182,* 776 (1973); *ibid. 183,* 258 (1974).

[84]George B. Hutchinson, "Causes of death with increasing rates in the 1960's," appendix A to the President's Science Advisory Committee, *Chemicals and Health,* 141-143 (1973).

precise and relevant interpretation to this measure, and about the approximations it involves, were it not true that other measures have, to greater or lesser degree, the same difficulties." Clearly there is a need for innovative work on these matters.

Because it is so difficult to gain an intuitive grasp of the magnitude of risks, especially those of great severity but very low probability, risks are often expressed in several ways and compared to classical or "natural" risks or to well-known technological risks, as an aid to comprehension. Several risk expressions were used in the recent Atomic Energy Commission-sponsored "Rasmussen report" (so called after the study director, Norman C. Rasmussen) on the accident risks of nuclear plants.

> From the viewpoint of a person living in the general vicinity of a reactor, the likelihood of being killed in any one year in a reactor accident is one chance in 300,000,000 and the likelihood of being injured in any one year in a reactor accident is one chance in 150,000,000. From a broader societal viewpoint, one individual of the 15 million people living in the vicinity of 100 reactors [the number of plants expected to be in use in the United States by about 1980] might be killed and 2 individuals might be injured every 25 years."

With regard to one of the most catastrophic types of nuclear plant disasters imaginable, "The most likely core melt accident would occur on the average of one every 17,000 years per plant." Further,

> If we consider a group of 100 similar plants then the chance of an accident causing 10 or more fatalities is 1 in 2500 per year or, on the average, one such accident every 25 centuries. For accidents involving 1000 or more fatalities the number is 1 in 1,000,000 or once in a million years. Interestingly, this is just the probability that a meteor would strike a U. S. population center and cause 1000 fatalities.

In comparison to other risks,

> The likelihood of reactor accidents is much smaller than many non-nuclear accidents having similar consequences. All non-nuclear accidents examined in this study, including fires, explosions, toxic chemical releases, dam failures, airplane crashes, earthquakes, hurricanes and tornadoes, are much more likely to occur and can have consequences comparable to or larger than nuclear accidents.

Any assessment of such an exceedingly complex technological problem requires making many assumptions and involves analytical methods whose very nature must be questioned. The Atomic Energy Commission report above should be consulted for details, as should the reviews and conflicting reports from other organizations.[85]

Often, the distribution of risks—over the population or over time—is as important as their magnitude. Summary risk figures become much more revealing when broken down by groups of victims. Thus there are implications for design and education in the fact that 17 percent of all portable electric fan injuries involve children under five years of age.[86] As to distribution over time, the social and political impact of a single catastrophe affecting many people at one time is usually greater than that of a chronic hazard affecting the same number of people just as seriously but over a long period.

[85]U. S. Atomic Energy Commission [U. S. Nuclear Regulatory Commission], *An Assessment of Accident Risks in U. S. Commercial Nuclear Power Plants*; the above quotations are from the summary volume, AEC no. WASH-1400 (August, 1974). Also see Sierra Club/Union of Concerned Scientists, Henry W. Kendall and Sidney Moglewer, preparors, *Preliminary Review of the AEC Reactor Safety Study* (November, 1974); U. S. Environmental Protection Agency, *Comments by the Environmental Protection Agency on reactor safety study: An Assessment of Accident Risks in U. S. Commercial Nuclear Power Plants,* (November, 1974).

[86]U. S. Consumer Product Safety Commission, "Portable electric fans," *NEISS News 3,* no. 1 (July, 1974).

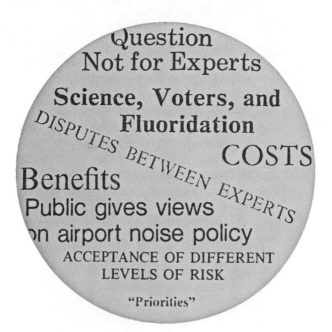

Question
Not for Experts
Science, Voters, and
Fluoridation

DISPUTES BETWEEN EXPERTS

COSTS

Benefits
Public gives views
on airport noise policy
ACCEPTANCE OF DIFFERENT
LEVELS OF RISK

"Priorities"

3

Judging Safety

Nowhere in the previous chapter did we mention "measuring safety." In fact, we deliberately avoided the word "safety" altogether, because of its vagueness and long history of misuse. Safety is not measured. *Risks* are measured. Only when those risks are weighed on the balance of social values can safety be judged: *a thing is safe if its attendant risks are judged to be acceptable.*

Determining safety, then, involves two extremely different kinds of activities; a prime objective of this text, and a critical obligation of those who make or study public decisions, is to emphasize the distinction:

Measuring risk—measuring the probability and severity of harm—is an empirical, scientific activity;

Judging safety—judging the acceptability of risks—is a normative, political activity.

Although the difference between the two would seem obvious, it is all too often forgotten, ignored, or obscured. This failing is often the cause of the disputes that hit the front pages.

We advocate use of this particular definition for many reasons. It encompasses the other, more specialized, definitions. By employing the word "acceptable" it emphasizes that safety decisions are relativistic and judgmental. It immediately elicits the crucial questions, "Acceptable in whose view?" and "Acceptable in what terms?" and "Acceptable for whom?" Further, it avoids all implication that safety is an intrinsic, absolute, measurable property of things.

In the following four examples, risk-measuring activity is described in Roman type, and safety-judging in italics.

- Shopping for a lawn-mower gasoline can, a man compares cans having explosion-proof "safety closures" with ones having ordinary lids. The safety cans cost a good deal more, but, bearing the seal of an independent testing laboratory, they are certified as less hazardous than other designs. *Put on guard by recent newspaper warnings about fuel can explosions, he judges the ordinary cans to be too risky for his family, despite their greater convenience and lower cost. He buys a safety can.*

- A legislature asks questions about seat belts: How effective are they? Will people wear them? What reduction in injuries can be expected from seat belts? How much do they cost? Can manufacturers make them available in all new cars? *How much does society value that injury reduction? Are the belts an acceptable solution? Should they be required by law?*

- A scientific advisory committee is charged by the government with recommending radiation exposure standards. The committee reviews all the animal experiments, the occupational medical record, the epidemiological surveys of physicians and patients exposed to X-rays, and the studies of the survivors of the Nagasaki and Hiroshima explosions. It inventories the modes of exposure; it reviews present radiation standards, including those of other nations and international organizations; and it examines the practical possibility of reducing exposures. *It weighs all the risks, costs, and benefits, and then decides that the allowed exposure has been unacceptably high; it recommends that because the intensity of some major sources, such as medical X-rays, can be reduced at reasonable cost and with little loss of effectiveness, the standards should be made more restrictive.*

- Over a three-year period, William Ruckelshaus, administrator of the Environmental Protection Agency, considered many different petitions from the various interested parties before acting on his agency's inquiry into the use of DDT. Finally, in 1972, he ruled that the scientific evidence led him to conclude that DDT is "an uncontrollable, durable chemical that persists in the aquatic and terrestrial environments" and "collects in the food chain," and that although the evidence regarding human tumorogenicity and other long-term effects was inconclusive, there was little doubt that DDT has serious ecological effects. Ruckelshaus reviewed the benefits of DDT in the protection of cotton and other crops and affirmed that other equally effective pesticides were available. *Summing the arguments, then, he ruled that "the long-range risks of continued use of DDT for use on cotton and most other crops is unacceptable and outweighs any benefits. ..."*[87]

The notion of acceptability is pervasive, although it is seldom given explicit emphasis (emphasis is supplied typographically in the following examples). In a report on the accident risks from nuclear power plants:

> While the study has presented the estimated risks from nuclear power plant accidents and compared them with other risks that exist in our society, it has made no judgment on the *acceptability* of nuclear risks. Although the study believes nuclear accident risks are very small, the judgment as to what level of risk society should *accept* is a broader one than can be made here.[88]

And in the title of a food supply report:

> A report on current ethical considerations in the determination of *acceptable* risk with regard to food and food additives.[89]

In heading down the slopes a skier attests that he accepts the risks; at a later stage of his life he may reject those very same risks because of

---

[87]U. S. Environmental Protection Agency, "Consolidated DDT hearings," *37 Federal Register,* 13369-13376 (July 7, 1972).

[88]U. S. Atomic Energy Commission, "An assessment of accident risks in U. S. commercial nuclear power plants," AEC no. WASH-1400, summary volume p. 7 (September, 1974).

[89]Citizens' Commission on Science, Law and the Food Supply (March 25, 1974).

changes in his awareness, his physical fragility, or his responsibilities to family or firm. While one woman may accept the side effects of oral contraceptives because she doesn't want to risk pregnancy, another woman may so fear the pill that she judges a diaphragm to be a more acceptable compromise among the several risks. Even though he is fully aware of the mangled fingers, chronic coughs, or damaged eyes or ears of those around him, a worker may accept those risks rather than endure the daily nuisance and tedium of blade guards, respirators, goggles, or ear protectors; but his employer, for reasons of cost, paternalism, or government requirement, may find this risky behavior unacceptable.

The elusive character of the word *acceptable* led a report on congressional radiation protection hearings to offer some guidance in "untangling the language of the record":

> 'Acceptable' is used to mean such different things as (a) a conscious decision perhaps based upon some balancing of good and bad or progress and risk, (b) a decision implying a comparison, possibly subjective, with hazards from other causes, these latter being 'acceptable' in turn in one of the senses given here, or perhaps just historically and possibly unconsciously, (c) the passive but substantive fact that nothing has been done to eliminate or curtail the thing being deemed 'acceptable.'[90]

Acceptance may be just a passive, or even stoical, continuance of historical momentum, as when people accept their lot at a dangerous traditional trade or continue to live near a volcano. Acceptance may persist because no alternatives are seen, as in the case of automobiles and many other technological hazards. Acceptance may result from ignorance or misperception of risk: variations on "I didn't know the gun was loaded" and "It won't happen to me" show up in every area. Acceptance may be simply acquiescence in a majority decision, such as a referendum-based decision on fluoridation, or in a decision by some governing elite, as with the average person's tacit approval of most public standards. Acceptance may even be an expression of preference for moderate but known risks over perhaps smaller but less well understood risks, as with preference for coal- and oil-fired power plants over nuclear plants. Later parts of this chapter will deal further with these points. For now, it is important to appreciate that such decisions may or may not be—and are certainly not necessarily—fair, just, consistent, efficient, or rational.

---

[90]U. S. Congress, Joint Committee on Atomic Energy, "Radiation protection criteria and standards: Their basis and use," Summary-analysis of hearings May 24-25 and June 1-3, 1960.

There is a great deal of overlap between the two decisionmaking domains implied by our definition of safety. Scientists, engineers, and medical people are called upon by political officials to judge the desirability of certain courses for society. Panels of scientists recommend exposure limits. Physicians prescribe medicines and diets. Engineers design dams, television sets, toasters, and airplanes. All of these decisions are heavily, even if only implicitly, value-laden.

On the other hand, by adopting particular risk data in their deliberations, political and judiciary agents at least implicitly rule on the correctness of measurements. The business of determining risk must often be settled operationally in hearings or other political deliberations, because the day-to-day management of society can't always wait for scientists to complete their cautious, precise determinations, which may take years. Congressional committees and regulatory agencies conduct hearings and issue rulings on the risks of food additives and air pollutants. Courts rule on the dangers of DDT. Risk and its acceptability are weighed by both manufacturers and consumers in the push-and-pull of the marketplace.

Between the two activities—measuring risk and judging safety—lies a discomforting no-man's-land ... or every-man's-land. Scientists on the fringe of the political arena, attempting to avoid charges of elitism, are looking for more objective ways to appraise society's willingness to accept various risks. At the same time, political officials confronted by scientifically controversial "facts" that never seem to gain the clarity promised by textbooks are exploring the possibilities of advisory assistance, fact-finding hearings, and formal technology assessments.

GUIDES TO ACCEPTABILITY

"Reasonableness." This is by far the most commonly cited and most unimpeachable principle in safety judgments. For instance, the legislative charter of the Consumer Product Safety Commission directs it to "reduce unreasonable risk of injury" associated with consumer goods.[91] Panels of experts frequently invoke a "rule of reason" in rendering advice. The concept of reasonableness pervades economic analyses of hazard reduction and the structures of legal liability.

Unfortunately, reference to reasonableness is in a sense a phantom citation. It provides little specific guidance for public decisionmakers, for whom reasonableness is presumably a requirement for staying in office.

---

[91]"Consumer Product Safety Act," *Public Law 92-573* (1972).

Not surprisingly, the Consumer Product Safety Act does not venture to define reasonableness. As guidance, the Safety Commission quotes the description given by the final report of its progenitor, the National Commission on Product Safety:

> Risks of bodily harm to users are not unreasonable when consumers understand that risks exist, can appraise their probability and severity, know how to cope with them, and voluntarily accept them to get benefits that could not be obtained in less risky ways. When there is a risk of this character, consumers have reasonable opportunity to protect themselves; and public authorities should hesitate to substitute their value judgments about the desirability of the risk for those of the consumers who choose to incur it.
>
> But preventable risk is not reasonable
>
> (a) when consumers do not know that it exists; or
>
> (b) when, though aware of it, consumers are unable to estimate its frequency and severity; or
>
> (c) when consumers do not know how to cope with it, and hence are likely to incur harm unnecessarily; or
>
> (d) when risk is unnecessary in ... that it could be reduced or eliminated at a cost in money or in the performance of the product that consumers would willingly incur if they knew the facts and were given the choice.[92]

The point of safety judgments is indeed to decide what is reasonable; it's just that any rational decision will have to be made on more substantive bases, such as the following, which are in a sense criteria for reasonableness.

Custom of usage. The Food and Drug Administration has designated hundreds of food additives as "generally recognized as safe" (GRAS). The GRAS list, established in 1958, includes such substances as table salt, vitamin A, glycerin, and baking powder, whose long use has earned them wide and generally unquestioned acceptance.[93] Being classified as GRAS exempts those substances from having to pass certain premarket clearances. From time to time this sanction is challenged, but most critics of the GRAS list have argued not so much that it should be abandoned as that individual items should be subjected to periodic review. In 1969, following its decision to ban the popular artificial sweetener cyclamate (until then GRAS), the

---

[92]National Commission on Product Safety, *Final Report,* 11 (1970).

[93]*21 U. S. Code of Federal Regulations,* 121.101 (subpart B).

Food and Drug Administration initiated a full review of the GRAS list. That review is still in progress, and "so far nothing has been found to lead to any further bans similar to the one on cyclamate."[94]

Prevailing professional practice. Long established as the criterion for physicians' clinical practice, this principle is increasingly being invoked in evaluating the protection that engineers, designers, and manufacturers provide their clients. Buildings are said to conform to the "prevailing local standards." Toys are "of a common design." X-ray machines are operated "at normal intensities." In many instances the wisdom of such deference to convention can be questioned. The underlying assumption is that if a thing has been in common use it must be okay, since any adverse effects would have become evident, and that a thing sanctioned by custom is safer than one not tested at all.

Best available practice, highest practicable protection, and lowest practicable exposure. Air and water quality regulations have stipulated that polluters control their emissions by the "best available means." So have noise abatement laws. Obviously, although such a requirement does provide the public regulator with a vague rationale, he must still exercise judgment over what constitutes "best" practice for every individual case and what economic factors should be considered in defining "practicable." Hardware for pollution control or noise abatement may exist, but only at a cost that many allege to be prohibitive; is it to be considered "available"?

Degree of necessity or benefit. This consideration was explicit in a statement from the 1969 White House Conference on Food, Nutrition and Health, which recommended that

> no additional chemicals should be permitted in or on foods unless they have been shown with reasonable certainty to be safe on the basis of the best scientific procedures available for the evaluation of safety and meet one or more of the following criteria:
>
> 1. They have been shown by appropriate tests to be significantly less toxic than food additives currently employed for the same purpose.
> 2. They significantly improve the quality or acceptability of the food.
> 3. Their use results in a significant increase in the food supply.

---

[94]Alan T. Spiher, Jr., "Food ingredient review: where it stands now," *FDA Consumer,* 23-26 (June 1974).

4. They improve the nutritive value of food.

5. Their use results in a decrease in the cost of food to the consumer.[95]

Similarly, the Environmental Mutagen Society has said:

> Given a reasonable calculation of the genetic hazard posed by an environmental mutagen, it then becomes necessary to consider how acceptable such a risk will be to the population at large. The guiding principle in all cases should be that no risk whatsoever is acceptable when the mutagenic compound presents no clear benefits, or when an alternative nonmutagenic compound is available.[96]

The Delaney principle. This principle, part of an amendment to the Food and Drug Act introduced in 1958 by Congressman James J. Delaney, requires that "no [food] additive shall be deemed to be safe if it is found . . . after tests which are appropriate for the evaluation of the safety of food additives to induce cancer in man or animal."[97]

Seemingly of the best intention—for who would wish to add proven carcinogens to anyone's food?—and seemingly a sharp decision tool for a regulator ("if it causes cancer, ban it"), this bold amendment has been controversial from the beginning. Because of the extraordinarily difficult problems of assessing carcinogenicity, as we described earlier, it is extremely difficult for either scientists or political officials to decide what "appropriate tests" are and what evidence suffices to prove that an agent can "induce cancer." Far from resolving the regulatory problem, the amendment has in some ways compounded it. The principle was intended to be an absolute, highly discriminating criterion, an aid to decision-making. But the Food and Drug Administration has used it as the explicit basis for decisions to ban fully registered products on only two occasions, both involving compounds used in food packaging materials. Nevertheless, the Delaney principle has served continually as a guide in many decisions even outside the area of foods. Its very existence, and the well-understood intentions behind it, are strong deterrents to risky actions. Indeed, some would like to see it extended to govern not only carcinogens but mutagens and teratogens as well; legislation to that effect has been pending in the

---

[95]*White House Conference on Food, Nutrition and Health, Final Report,* 130 (1970).

[96]Environmental Mutagen Society, committee 17, "Environmental mutagenic hazards," *Science 187,* 503-514 (1975).

[97]*21 U. S. Code of Federal Regulations* 409 (c)(3)(A); section 512 (d)(1)(H) extends the principle to animal-growth-promoting feed additives, and section 706 (b)(5)(B) to food colorings.

Congress, and petitions opposing and supporting such legislation are being circulated among scientists. Consumerist James Turner has stated that:

> The loose collection of organizations and individuals generally called the 'consumer movement' in the United States tends to believe that the principle of social policy embodied in the Delaney Clause is the best way to deal with these slower acting and less direct causes of death and chronic sickness. In general they are also highly skeptical that any better principle for dealing with the chemical threat to man can be found.[98]

Others, such as a panel of the President's Science Advisory Committee, have objected that the clause nullifies case-by-case judgments of risks, costs, and benefits:

> The rigid stipulation of the Delaney Clause, springing from presently inadequate biological knowledge, places the administrator in a very difficult interpretative position. He is not allowed, for example, to weigh any known benefits to human health, no matter how large, against the possible risks of cancer production, no matter how small.[99]

Some people object to singling out carcinogenic food additives for this special attention, which is not given to agents possibly causing liver disease, brain damage, or other serious disabilities. The debate continues. As scientists perfect techniques allowing detection of ever tinier amounts of chemicals, the viability of the Delaney principle will be challenged further. An impasse seems avoidable. Even now there are chemicals widely present in our food that are both detectable (using special techniques not necessarily employed on a routine basis) and carcinogenic (in some large dosage, under some conditions, to some particular test animal), but which are allowed to remain there by license of administrative oversight or bureaucratic definition as not being food additives or by invocation of a side-stepping "rule of reason."[100]

---

[98]James Turner, "Consumer views of the Delaney Amendment," in *Hearings before the House Agriculture—Environmental, and Consumer Protection Committee, Part 8, 225* (May 6, 1974).

[99]President's Science Advisory Committee, Panel on Chemicals and Health, *Chemicals and Health,* 11 (1973).

[100]Arguments have appeared in *Preventive Medicine 2,* 123-170 (1973), a special issue devoted to the Delaney Clause; in the President's Science Advisory Committee, *Chemicals and Health* (1973); in National Academy of Sciences/National Research Council, *How Safe is Safe? The Design of Policy on Drugs and Food Additives* (1974); and in the Food and Drug Administration, "Study of the Delaney clause and other anti-cancer clauses," *Hearings before the House Subcommittee on Agriculture—Environmental and Consumer Protection, Part 8* (May 6, 1974).

"No detectable adverse effect." Although such a principle is applied frequently in our everyday lives, and although it has a certain operational value, it is a weak criterion which may amount to little more than an admission of uncertainty or ignorance. Many hazards now recognized, such as moderate levels of X-rays or asbestos or vinyl chloride, could at an earlier time have been said to have "no detectable adverse effect."

"Toxicologically insignificant levels." On occasion, guidelines have been proposed under which toxicologically insignificant levels would be defined administraively for certain classes of food substances: chemicals which have been in sustained commercial production without evidence of toxicological hazard; pesticide degradation products occurring at very low levels; or chemicals about which toxicological information is lacking but which possess certain chemical structural features. This has been defended as a practical approach, but it is open to criticism as being quite arbitrary. One scientific panel has said that the concept of toxicologically insignificant dose levels, "of dubious merit in any life science, has absolutely no validity in the field of carcinogenesis" and has proposed alternative ways of establishing a "socially acceptable level of risk."[101]

The threshold principle. If it can be proven that there is indeed a level of exposure below which no adverse effect occurs, subthreshold exposures might be considered safe. But determining whether there really is a threshold, for the especially vulnerable as well as for the average populace, is usually a nearly impossible task. As we mentioned earlier, for loud noises there are clearly thresholds of annoyance, pain, and ear damage. But whether there are thresholds for effects of radiation, chemical carcinogens, and mutagens has never been firmly established.

EMPIRICAL CRITERIA OF ACCEPTABILITY

The above general guidelines are usefully supplemented by several empirical criteria.

---

[101]National Academy of Sciences/National Research Council, Food Protection Committee, *Guidelines for estimating toxicologically insignificant levels of chemicals in food* (1969); Ad Hoc Committee on the Evaluation of Low Levels of Environmental Chemical Carcinogens, "Evaluation of environmental carcinogens, Report to the Surgeon General, U. S. Public Health Service," in the *Congressional Record,* E952-958 (February 9, 1972).

Exposure relative to natural background. Following long precedent in radiation protection, the National Research Council's panel on the biological effects of radiation, to which we referred earlier, stated:

> Our first recommendation is that the natural background radiation be used as a standard for comparison. If the genetically significant exposure is kept well below this amount, we are assured that the additional consequences will neither differ in kind from those which we have experienced throughout human history nor exceed them in quantity.[102]

Although by itself this approach is not very substantial, as one of several complementary inputs to the standards-setting process it has proven very useful. Similar reasoning can be applied to other agents, such as noise, lead, and food ingredients, whose "natural background" levels are essentially irreducible. For each of these the background presence has served as a benchmark. But notice that unless one is willing to assume that Nature is perfectly benevolent, this argument should not be carried too far.

Occupational exposure precedent. From the 1713 publication of Bernardino Ramazzini's *De Morbis Artificum* ("Diseases of Workers") through the present, the experience of workers has given us valuable information about prolonged exposure.[103] In standards-setting, the occupational record is usually consulted for an indication of maximal exposure without ill effect; applying a generous "safety factor" to that figure then establishes a limit for the general public. As the young nuclear industry grew after the war, medical experience led to the adoption of occupational radiation standards. Workers' exposure was closely monitored. By the mid-1950s large numbers of people were being exposed to many sources and kinds of radiation, both on and off the job, and limits for non-occupational exposure became necessary. In 1956 both the National Council on Radiation Protection and the International Commission on Radiation Protection recommended that for the general public, exposure should be limited to no more than one-tenth the occupational levels.[104] (In this case, as in many others, the esthetically neat factor one-tenth is apparently an arbitrary selection; the factor one-eleventh is never chosen.)

---

[102]National Academy of Sciences/National Research Council, *The Effect on Populations of Exposure to Low Levels of Ionizing Radiation,* 113 (1972); this report was summarized on p. 42ff of this book.

[103]See English translation by Wilmer Cave Wright (Hafner Publishing Co., N. Y., 1964).

[104]Jacob Shapiro, *Radiation Protection,* 225 (Harvard University Press, Cambridge, 1972)

Public referenda and polling. These procedures have been applied in only a few instances, mostly in cases in which public interest is intense and in which people experience the hazard in an immediate, personal way, as with noise. In many cities, public referendum has been used to settle the issue of public water fluoridation. In this still controversial issue, it is difficult to evaluate the effectiveness of the referendum procedure compared to other administrative decision processes. Fluoridation offers one of the few examples of a widespread, direct community vote on a well-defined technological issue.[105]

People's subjective ratings of noises can be analyzed, as can lawsuits and annoyance complaints filed with civil authorities. Such analyses can correlate annoyance with factors of socioeconomic status, fear, importance of the noisy activities, perception of fair treatment, and the extent to which the noise can be controlled or reduced. Polling the public's willingness to accept various levels of noise has been important for setting standards, designing equipment and home products, and for planning and managing airports and communities.[106]

Comparison with accustomed hazards. This approach has been explored analytically, but so far it has been used very little, except quite casually, in making political decisions. It would assess people's attitudes about the risks attending travel, work, natural disaster, and communicable disease, and then use this information as a calibration for predicting attitudes toward new hazards. The technique shows promise but is still a long way from practical usefulness.[107]

AN ARRAY OF CONSIDERATIONS

Quite often it is useful to describe hazards by seeing how they fall within an array of considerations such as Figure 3-1.

---

[105]Harvey M. Sapolsky, "Science, voters, and the fluoridation controversy," *Science 162,* 427-433 (1969).

[106]Environmental Protection Agency, *Public Health and Welfare Criteria for Noise* (1973); Environmental Protection Agency, *Community Noise,* 50-79 (1971).

[107]Chauncey Starr, "Benefit-cost studies in sociotechnical systems," in National Academy of Engineering, *Perspectives on Benefit-Risk Decision Making,* 17-42 (1972); commentary on the Starr approach appears in Gilbert F. White, editor, *Natural Hazards: Local, National, Global* (Oxford University Press, 1975).

Figure 3-1. An array of considerations influencing safety judgments

Risk assumed voluntarily	Risk borne involuntarily
Effect immediate	Effect delayed
No alternatives available	Many alternatives available
Risk known with certainty	Risk not known
Exposure is an essential	Exposure is a luxury
Encountered occupationally	Encountered non-occupationally
Common hazard	"Dread" hazard
Affects average people	Affects especially sensitive people
Will be used as intended	Likely to be misused
Consequences reversible	Consequences irreversible

Risk assumed voluntarily	Risk borne involuntarily

As Chauncey Starr so memorably expressed it, "We are loath to let others do unto us what we happily do to ourselves."[108] Our opinions of what is acceptable definitely depend on the degree to which we are free to opt for or decline the risk. It is one thing to choose to go skiing, drive a sports car, use a tool without safeguards, smoke cigarettes, or eat the

[108]National Academy of Engineering, *Perspectives on Benefit-Risk Decision Making,* 30 (1972).

vegetables we have sprayed ourselves; but it is quite another to breathe the air and endure the noise where we live (and few of us are really free to move away), dodge the traffic on our way to work, or drink water from our municipal supply. For some purposes it may be useful to think of three categories: "individual or voluntary risks ..., risks where the individual's options are somewhat limited by social or governmental action ..., and risks in which governmental action preempts voluntary individual decision making."[109] According to most conceptions of regulatory control, risks that citizens have to bear involuntarily are the ones the government has the greatest responsibility to regulate: urban traffic and noise; the quality of the air and drinking water; and bridges, dams, power transmission lines, and other public works.

Effect immediate ——————————————— **Effect delayed**

We have emphasized the importance of this distinction repeatedly. Some hazards, such as arsenic, have both immediate and chronic (long-range) effects, with the proportion of the two kinds of effects determined by the nature and intensity of exposure.

No alternatives ——————————— **Many alternatives**
available **available**

If no practical alternatives are in sight, people seem to accept conditions, perhaps grudgingly or fatalistically; witness those who live in polluted industrial centers where "smoke is money" and the chances for change are slight. At the other extreme are household appliances, toys, toiletries, and other cases in which a profusion of competing products lets us be very choosy; at least indirectly (by not buying) and sometimes directly, we may chide a manufacturer for not adopting the safety features of his competitors' products. Major public decisions to ban certain pesticides (DDT) and food additives ("red food dye #2") have cited the availability of alternatives as part of the rationale for doing away with those agents.

Risk known ——————————— **Risk not**
with certainty **known**

How certain we are about risks influences our decisions strongly. In some cases well-known risks are preferred to lesser but unfamiliar

---

[109]National Academy of Engineering, *Perspectives on Benefit-Risk Decision Making,* 2 (1972).

ones; this especially happens when poorly appreciated new technologies are being introduced, or when a culture is apprehensively undergoing rapid change.

A recent analysis hybridized this factor with the preceding one in saying that:

We need to separate four classes of situations quite clearly:

- Situations where alternative suppliers offer the consumer very different quality for very different safety [detergents].
- Situations where all sources of supply provide an equivalent product whose dangers have been more or less widely understood for a long time [automobiles].
- Situations where all sources of supply provide an equivalent product whose dangers have only recently been confirmed [cigarettes].
- Situations where all sources of supply provide an equivalent product whose safety is open to some question, but where there is no established danger [mercury-tainted swordfish].[110]

Exposure is		**Exposure is**
an	———————————	**a**
essential		**luxury**

Clearly our appraisal of any risk is influenced by the extent to which exposure to it is necessary. This criterion may be given more importance in coming years as we learn more about individuals' overall physiological burdens. It is likely that some luxuries in which we now indulge, such as cigarettes and certain cosmetics and food additives, will in the future be judged unnecessarily taxing to our bodies. While aspirin will probably keep its place in our medicine cabinets, barbiturates may suffer the same banishment that household codeine did a few years ago.

Encountered	———————————	**Encountered**
occupationally		**non-occupationally**

It has traditionally been accepted that pursing one's trade will almost inevitably bring a peculiar set of risks, and further, that such risks may allowably be greater than for non-occupational activities. This attitude

---

[110]President's Science Advisory Committee, Panel on Chemicals and Health, *Chemicals and Health,* 119 (1973).

89

has strong historical momentum. The justification has been that "taking those chances is what you get paid for." A coal miner, a housewife, a stevedore, a truck driver, a desk-bound office worker, and a farmer all expect certain hazards. Although people have always tried to reduce their work hazards, systematic effort has been made only in recent years, and even then, in just a few prosperous nations. In part this is due to a new general awareness and apprehension about subtle, chronic hazards such as noise, asbestos, and vinyl chloride. In part it is a manifestation of the recent years' redistribution of social rights and power. It is a relatively new development that society as a whole should show concern for the conditions in the mines and foundries, or that society would offer to underwrite (as taxes, or as consumer costs) the alleviation of suffering in chemical plants and textile mills. As indications of a remarkable change in attitude we should point not just to the dramatic crusades over asbestosis and black lung, but also to the development of orthopedically correct tractor seats, eye-saving standards for factory lighting, and quieter garbage trucks.

However, our attitudes about risks and our assignment of responsibility for minimizing them still seem to be influenced by whether they are encountered on or off the job. Comparing the air pollutant standards set for protection of the general public by the Environmental Protection Agency (EPA) with those for workers set by the Labor Department's Occupational Safety and Health Administration (OSHA) (see Table 3-1), environmentalist Barry Commoner has concluded that "it would appear, then, that in absolute terms the two sets of standards require that the worker accept an environmental insult which is not tolerated outside the workplace." The reasons for this are many and difficult to analyze (several are pointed out by Commoner in his article), but the generalization seems true.[111]

Pursuit of occupation is still distinct from other activities, despite recent idealistic exhortations that work be indistinguishably integrated with the rest of our daily affairs. Some nations, such as the Soviet Union, have endorsed formal policies with the goal that workers should be at no greater risk in carrying out their labor than they are off the job. Admirable though such a goal is, it has probably never been very closely approached in any country.[112]

[111]Barry Commoner, "Workplace burden," Environment 15, no. 6, 15-20 (1973).

[112]Harold J. Magnuson, "Soviet and American standards for industrial health," Archives of Environmental Health 10, 542-545 (1965). Harold J. Magnuson, David W. Fassett, Horace W. Gerarde, Verald K. Rowe, Henry F. Smythe, Jr., and Herbert E. Stokinger, "Industrial toxicology in the Soviet Union — theoretical and applied," American Industrial Hygiene Association Journal 25, 185-197 (1964).

**Table 3-1. Environmental versus Occupational Standards
for Selected Air Pollutants***

Pollutant	Environmental Standard (EPA)	Occupational Standard (OSHA)
Sulfur dioxide[a] (annual arithmetic mean)	0.03 ppm[b]	5 ppm
Carbon monoxide (max. 8 hr. once/year[a])	9 ppm	50 ppm
Nitrogen dioxide (annual arithmetic mean)	0.5 ppm	5 ppm
Particulates (respirable fraction, annual arithmetic mean)	0.075 mg/m^{3C}	5 mg/m^3

Common hazard ———————————————— **"Dread" hazard**

Some hazards are met with an almost stoical acceptance. We seem resigned to the recurrence of some accidents: children just will have those scrapes, bruises, and broken arms, kitchens will have fires, and bicycle riders will have to take their knocks. This is not to say that those accidents are not regrettable or anguishing—they most certainly are. However, that response can be distinguished from the sort of inordinate dread or horror that might attend news of the accidental death of a child, the grisly mangling of a machine operator, or sickness from a silent, invisible beam of radiation. Again, these are all deplorable. But for various reasons each has about it an overtone of dread that may attract publicity and official attention out of proportion to its overall risk to society. This is not necessarily bad; it may catalyze action in other areas or set an important precedent. It can, however, skew public opinion, garner high priority for the prevention of some highly improbable event, and thereby reduce priorities for preventing less dramatic but serious and more probable hazards, to the detriment of the overall health of the population.

[a]Ambient air standards are given several values for short-term concentrations: that is, "maximum n-hour concentration not to be exceeded more than once per year." All in-plant exposures are presumably for an eight-hour day.

[b]Parts per million.

[c]Milligrams per cubic meter.

*Adapted from Barry Commoner, *Environment 15*, no. 6, 19 (1973).

Affects
average ————————————————————
people

Affects
especially sensitive
people

Some controversies over detergents have centered upon protecting allergic people, as have disputes over ragweed eradication campaigns and over cosmetics. (What should constitute "hypoallergenic" cosmetics?) A British scientist, charging that his country's noise laws don't protect the sensitive, has recently argued that "one-fifth of the population are far more sensitive to noise than planners assume, while another third aren't bothered at all. Only the rest are 'average.' "[113] This consideration is important in decisions about every publicly-managed hazard. Scientifically, it is exceedingly difficult to gauge how sensitivities range through a large population. Politically, public officials are understandably reluctant to admit that a decision on a problem will protect only, say, 99 percent of the American population; even protecting 99.99 percent of a 225,000,000-person nation still leaves 22,500 people at risk. Given the amazing ways in which human beings differ from each other, it seems highly unlikely that such measures as environmental, occupational, and consumer safety regulation can ever in fact guarantee "equal protection of all Americans" as some well-meant but naive legislations proclaim. At the least, however, safety decisions should consider what proportion of those exposed are to be protected.

Will be used as intended ————————————— **Likely to be misused**

Designers, engineers, manufacturers, the government, purchasers, and guardians of the very young and the senile all need to anticipate the degree to which products are likely to be misused. Tools must be designed for rugged use. Safeguards have to be built into products to protect the sleepy, the unwary, the immature, the aged, and the uneducated. Managers of workplaces must anticipate the carelessness that comes from long, dulling familiarity with a monotonous, repetitive task. Food processors have to think of the over-eaters and those with idiosyncratic food preferences. Purchasers need to be concerned for their families and for others who may be exposed to household products. Whose responsibility is it to anticipate misuse? To what extent should society pay the price for devising and building in protection for the relatively few who misuse products? These considerations are important, for instance, in the current debate over whether the Consumer Product Safety Commission should require that all

---

[113]Michael Bryan, "Noise laws don't protect the sensitive," *New Scientist*, 738-740 (September 27, 1973).

mattresses for sale be fire-retardant in order to protect the small fraction of the public who smoke in bed (and their families and neighbors). In some cases misuse may be the most important precipitating cause of accident, as it is for the thousands of astonished and often badly injured people who walk through glass doors every year.

Consequences reversible ———————————— Consequences irreversible

If the adverse effects eventually turn out to be worse than expected, can the situation be "undone," the agent retrieved, the consequences reversed? This has been an important consideration in the decision in the United States to ban such persistent agents as DDT which, once released into the environment, may spread irretrievably through air, water, and flesh, to disintegrate only much later.[114] In the pesticide case, other chemicals having greater cost and in many cases greater acute toxicity, but shorter lives, have been deemed preferable; at least if they ambush us they won't last long. Such a factor may be critical in forthcoming decisions about the aerosol-propellant freons, plutonium and other deadly waste from the nuclear industry, and other widely dispersed, persistent environmental hazards, and about agents that are suspected of human mutagenic effect.

Notice how the above categorizations differentiate between the following two examples. Snowmobiles are principally luxury products designed for average users who voluntarily employ them for recreational transportation, even though alternatives are available. They are associated with accidents, often from misuse but occasionally from mechanical failure, having the immediate and well-known consequences common to impact accidents. In addition, for frequent and unusually sensitive users they may have the delayed effect of impairing hearing. They may of course harm non-users as well. (It has been estimated that the one-and-one-half-million snowmobiles in the United States were associated with more than 19,000 hospital emergency room admissions during 1973.)[115]

To give a quite different example, nuclear power plants are thought to be essential by those who believe that the alternative ways of generating power will not meet the demands. For the general public, the risks are inescapable once these expensive plants are in operation. What the risks really are is quite controversial. The risks will be both to those who work

---

[114]See Chapter 6, "DDT: An archetypal modern problem."

[115]U. S. Consumer Product Safety Commission, *Fact Sheet No. 27: Snowmobiles* (July, 1974).

in the plants and to the general public. Effects will be both immediate, in the event of a catastrophic accident, and delayed, with any radiation exposures. There is a possibility, even if slight, of misuse such as sabotage. Both the radiation hazards and the unlikely-but-horrible explosion hazards carry overtones of dread.

Describing hazards in terms of this array of considerations can often help clarify the nature of problems and make explicit what the public debate is all about.

DECISIONS, DECISIONS, DECISIONS

Whether they are made systematically or haphazardly, deliberately or casually, by individuals or by institutions, decisions comprise several fundamental components which are apposed, compared, and weighed against each other. The following four are essentially matters of empirical fact.

Risk is a measure of the probability and severity of adverse effects.

Efficacy is a corresponding measure of the probability and intensity of beneficial effects.

Cost would seem only too familiar a measure. In recent years, however, there has been a move to broaden the usage of "cost" to include not just financial burden but all that must be paid in terms of manpower, material resources, social options, individual freedom, and other goods. Since much of this redefinition has been prompted by a new awareness of our relation to our worldly environment, it is hardly out of place to cite Henry David Thoreau's definition in *Walden*: "The cost of a thing is the amount of what I will call life which is required to be exchanged for it, immediately or in the long run." For many purposes cost includes not only final manufacturing, installation, operating, and maintenance costs but also development costs, legal transaction costs, regulatory costs, and the costs of opportunities precluded. Some costs may be "externalized"—that is, excluded in the accounting from the point of view of some benefited party. For example, industrial pollution may impose high health and other costs on a community but not cost the polluter or his customers anything. By contrast, part of the costs of industrial accidents may be internalized with the corporation in the form of insurance costs and be passed on to consumers and stockholders. Assessing the costs of technologies which are deeply embedded in the structure of society may be nearly impossible. Further, there will always be such intangibles as peace of mind (as affected, for instance, by noise),

94

the stability of the job market (as affected by government regulation of occupational safety), and the general quality of life.

Distribution of risks, benefits, and costs may be a political issue, but in many senses it is still an empirical matter. Who will end up paying? Will those who benefit be the ones paying? Will those at risk be the ones to benefit? Often the answers can be surveyed or estimated.

Appraising the above empirical factors generates the following derivative characterizations, which are matters of personal and social value judgment.

Safety is the degree to which risks are judged acceptable.

Benefit is the degree to which efficacies are judged desirable.

Equity of distribution of risks, benefits, and costs is a judgment of fairness and social justice.[116]

The above notions are logically symmetrical: *safety* is to *risk* as *benefit* is to *efficacy*. Risk and efficacy are matters of measurable, empirical fact; safety and benefit are matters of value judgment.

Empirical	Normative
Risk	Safety
Efficacy	Benefit
Distribution of hazards, benefits, and costs	Equity of distribution of hazards, benefits, and costs

Just as risk can be measured scientifically, so can efficacy. In recent years the efficacy of prescription drugs has been under intense review. The 1962 Kefauver-Harris amendments to the Food, Drug and Cosmetic Act require manufacturers to furnish proof that their new products are efficacious as well as safe—that is, that they not only are of acceptable risk but are sufficiently effective at accomplishing their therapeutic purpose. The Food and Drug Administration's review of efficacy studies carried out by the National Research Council has found that a large number of the first 900 drugs studied were unacceptably ineffective. These reviews, which will have great economic, legal, and therapeutic

---

[116]John Rawls, *Theory of Justice* (Harvard University Press, Cambridge, 1971); Norman Daniels, editor, *Reading Rawls* (Basic Books, Inc., N.Y., 1975); Victor Fuchs, *Who Shall Live?* (Basic Books, Inc., N.Y., 1974); Arthur M. Okun, *Equality and Efficiency: The Big Trade-Off* (Brookings Institution, Washington, D.C., 1975).

impact, are still being completed and are the subject of continuing debate.[117]

Strong controversy has recently arisen over diagnostic X-rays. One question is, "In view of the radiation hazards and rapidly rising costs of medical care, are physicians using too many X-rays?" Efficacy studies are providing helpful data. A study in Seattle has attempted to "discover the current information yield of skull series taken for injury" and to "determine if there is some rational strategy for selecting for skull radiographs only the patients who have a definite likelihood of being benefited by the procedure." Classifying 1500 patients into two groups identified a high-yield group of 1065 examinations that had revealed 92 fractures, and a low-yield group of 435 examinations that had revealed among them only one fracture. This led the investigators, themselves physicians, to conclude that "X-ray examination in the latter group could have been deferred or omitted without adverse effect on the patient's medical care ... We question whether physicians will be successful in defending against their critics standards of patient selection in which 20 percent of skull radiographs are performed for trivial injury or in which 34 percent are performed for primarily medicolegal reasons or in which 50 percent are performed with the estimation that there is only one chance in 100 of finding a fracture, with a true yield of one in 378."[118]

It may eventually prove possible to evaluate benefit systematically, but so far this has been done even less well than with safety. However, the corresponding primary attribute—efficacy—is more manageable, and it urgently deserves to be developed as a policymaking tool. Perhaps benefit analysis will follow.

The skull X-ray case illustrates how evaluations might proceed. First, the agent's efficacy is estimated. (*How successful is the diagnostic technique at revealing skull fractures?*) Next, the benefits of such efficacy are judged. (*What are the benefits of such diagnosis to the injured persons? To society?*) Then the distribution of the benefits is surveyed. (*What patients are affected? What benefits, such as protection from malpractice claims, accure to physicians in using the X-rays?*) A similar progression of

---

[117]National Academy of Sciences/National Research Council, *Drug Efficacy Study, Final Report* (1969); Roberta G. Marks, "Pharmaceuticals," in *The Legislation of Product Safety*, vol. 2, Samuel S. Epstein and Richard D. Grundy, editors, 143-196 (MIT Press, Cambridge, 1974); and Judith Axler Turner, "FDA pursues historic role amid public, industry pressures," *National Journal Reports*, 250-259 (February 15, 1975).

[118]Russell S. Bell and John W. Loop, "The utility and futility of radiographic skull examination for trauma," *The New England Journal of Medicine 284*, 236-239 (1971).

judgments fills in the other side of the ledger. Risks are measured. (*What are the risks from the radiation exposure? What might be the risks of not using the procedure?*) Safety is judged. (*Are the risks of a type and magnitude that the public is generally willing to accept?*) The distribution of the hazards is surveyed. (*What are the risks to the patients? To the radiologists and technicians?*) The costs are appraised, as is their distribution. An evaluation is built up, starting with measurable characteristics and progressing through more values-sensitive ones. All the above factors are weighed on what we have referred to as "the balance of social values." Corresponding characteristics of alternative agents are compared. Eventually an overall decision is made to manufacture, buy, regulate, prohibit, or take other action.

One way to envision balancing benefit and safety is the following. Suppose that a new drug has been tested clinically. Curve *A* in Figure 3-2 plots the percentage of people benefited (in some defined way) relative to the dose administered. Curve *B* plots the percentage of people affected adversely. In this first, too-good-to-be-true hypothetical case, the safe but efficacious dose is obviously about 10 units, where the greatest efficacy is secured at the lowest risk.

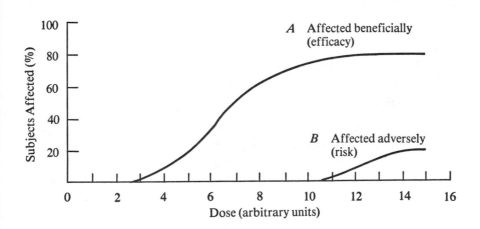

Figure 3-2. Relation of administered dose to percentage of subjects affected beneficially (A) and adversely (B): first case.

In a second (here-comes-real-life) case, suppose the curves run as shown in Figure 3-3. If *A* here is some lifesaving effect and *B* a lesser effect such as hives, the optimal dosage against serious disease might be roughly 12 units, in order to ensure efficacious treatment; a few patients would just have to tolerate the hives. But if the agent under examination is not a lifesaving drug but a suntan lotion, and *A* is protection against sunburn and *B* is causing hives, the optimal dosage probably would be judged as 7 or 8 units. In making these decisions we are, at least informally, assigning values to the efficacies and risks, subjectively translating them into benefit and safety. We do this in many areas every day, both individually and as a society.

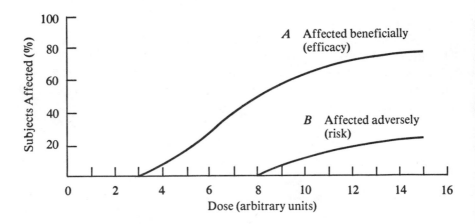

Figure 3-3. Relation of administered dose to percentage of subjects affected beneficially (A) and adversely (B): second case.

The components of summary decisions can often be "factored out" and appraised independently before the larger decisions are made. The safety of several things can often be compared without reference to cost, efficacy, or other variables. For instance, we can determine with full assurance that a third-wire-grounded power drill, whatever its extra cost or inconvenience, is safer with respect to electrical hazard than one that isn't grounded. Comparing "the Pill" with the IUD, one can ask which is less expensive to buy and administer, which presents less risk to health, and which is more efficacious at preventing pregnancy—and then decide which is preferable in the particular situation.

Society is now challenged by problems that have escalated beyond intuitive common-sense management. What really are the relative desirabilities of the various methods for treating heroin addiction or mental illness, for generating electricity, or for controlling world population growth? In tooling up for these problems, serious efforts are being made to bring order and rigor to the decision process. The approaches referred to as "risk-benefit analysis" try to quantify as many variables as possible and then calculate the balance or optimum for the situation. No matter what assumptions they embrace, such analyses are still at best comparisons of incommensurables—deaths and dollars, tumors and kilowatt-hours—and can hardly place proper values on integrity of community, personal grief, missed opportunity, beauty of surroundings, or the preciousness of the human hereditary material.

All reservations aside, we *do* make such judgments, even if clumsily, and we will have to continue to make them. Careful analyses can be quite useful in organizing widely dispersed and previously unreviewed information, identifying intangibles, and establishing grounds for rational comparison. Alternatives can be laid out and issues given shape. Unpromising alternatives can be rejected. Even if it does not in itself solve the problem, stating the issues clearly can aid in projecting the less obvious consequences of the options. Further, when particular analyses are endorsed or acknowledged by public officials, they become instruments for securing public disclosure of the bases for the decisions, bases that might otherwise remain undisclosed and unexamined.

In practice so far, risk-benefit analyses have been used mostly as background information. The art is so primitive that in debates, differing analyses can simply be played off against each other. For an official who refers to himself as being "on the firing line" or "in the hot seat," a lengthy, detailed, formal analysis whose very opening assumptions ("for purposes of analysis the value of a life is taken to be $250,000") are untuitively unsettling and open to challenge may just not find use, unless it happens to substantiate opinions arrived at by other means.[119]

---

[119]Lester B. Lave and Warren E. Weber, "A benefit-cost analysis of auto safety features," *Applied Economics 10*, 265-275 (1970); Lester B. Lave and Eugene P. Seskin, "Air Pollution and human health," *Science 169*, 723-733 (1970); National Academy of Engineering, *Perspectives on Benefit-Risk Decision Making* (1972); Henry D. Jacoby, John D. Steinbrunner, and others, *Clearing the Air: Federal Policy on Automotive Emission Control* (Ballinger, Cambridge, 1973); U. S. Environmental Protection Agency, *The Quality of Life Concept. A Potential New Tool for Decision Makers (1973)*; John Dunster, "Costs and benefits of nuclear power," *New Scientist*, 192-194 (October 18, 1973); National Academy of Sciences/National Academy of Engineering, *Air quality and automotive emission control*, prepared for the U. S. Senate Committee on Public Works (September, 1974), see especially vol. 4, "The costs and benefits of automobile pollution control."

Some public deliberations stretch the definition so much that they probably shouldn't be thought of as risk-benefit decisions at all. With problems that have disturbing uncertainty about them, we may choose a cautious course so as to spare ourselves even the possibility of surprise. For example, such an attitude has in part underlain opposition to the supersonic transport aircraft (SST). For many, the important considerations are not so much the SST's known risks (of the sort possessed by existing airplanes, only greater), their known, enormous costs (of development, manufacture, and maintenance), their known efficacies (high work capacity and flight speeds), or their known benefits (fast long-distance transportation), but rather the unknown risks (Will the sonic boom impair people's hearing, disturb their sleep, induce psychiatric illness? Will polluting the upper atmosphere increase skin cancer, change the climate? Could that damage be reversed?) and unknown costs (of noise suppression, of redesigning airports, of health and environmental damage).[120] To be sure, economic and other factors have been dominant in the SST debate. But so far the dictum, "If in doubt, don't," has also prevailed. In this and other instances, such as the upper-atmosphere ozone problem, the argument is not so much a true balancing of risks against benefits as it is an anguishing over uncertainty itself.

Some problems seem hardly amenable to technical solution. Biologist Garrett Hardin has provocatively drawn attention to what he calls the "tragedy of the commons," referring to a situation in which herdsmen, each trying to maximize his own gain, graze their animals on their village's commons. Overgrazing leads to ruin for all. The only solution for such problems, in which allocation by private demand overtaxes a collective resource, would seem to be "mutual coercion mutually agreed upon." The world now has become so complex, with resources limited and parts greatly interdependent, that just such a tragedy is unfolding with such problems as population growth and environmental pollution. Whether such grave problems indeed have technical solutions is an important question, and whether humankind will be able to devise workable political solutions in time remains to be seen.[121]

---

[120]Joel Primack and Frank von Hippel, *Advice and Dissent: Scientists in the Political Arena*, 10-29 (Basic Books, New York, 1974).

[121]Garrett Hardin, "The tragedy of the commons," *Science 162*, 1243-1248 (1968); commentary on Hardin's thesis is presented by Beryl L. Crowe, "The tragedy of the commons revisited," *Science 166*, 1103-1107 (1969), and by Thomas C. Schelling, "On the ecology of micromotives," *The Public Interest* no. 25, 59-98 (1971); the notion is applied to the health arena in Howard H. Hiatt, "Protecting the medical commons: who is responsible?" *New England Journal of Medicine 293*, 235-241 (1975).

Alvin Weinberg has argued that for problems attended by great uncertainty or having strong political overtones, adequate solutions cannot be supplied by science alone; he terms these problems "trans-scientific." He gives as examples the practical impossibility of assessing precisely the biological effects of radiation (because, short of experimenting on billions of mice or many people, our estimates will remain quite uncertain) and determining the probability of extremely improbable events such as earthquake destruction of Hoover Dam or a catastrophic nuclear reactor accident (because never in either case will we deliberately do the experiment). Weinberg emphasizes that the solving of such problems is as much a political activity as a scientific one.[122]

The notions of the "tragedy of the commons" and "trans-scientific problems" need to be explored. Are they valid, and if so, what are their implications for action?

---

[122]Alvin M. Weinberg, "Science and trans-science," *Minerva 10,* 209-222 (1972); Alvin M. Weinberg, "Science and trans-science," *Science 177,* 211 (1972); for commentary see Harvey Brooks, "Science and trans-science," *Minerva 10,* 484-486 (1972). Also see Wolf Häfele, "Hypotheticality and the new challenges: The pathfinder role of nuclear energy," *Minerva 12,* 303-322 (1974).

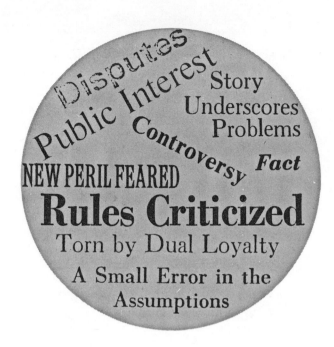

4

Safety Issues as Public Problems

The preceding chapters presented the conceptual principles without making special reference to the people and institutions using them, saying very little about who measures risks, judges safety, or takes safeguarding action. We now turn to the questions of who does what, where responsibilities lie, and how controversies arise, develop, and run their courses.

FROM QUIET TO CRISIS, AND BACK

A public problem arises with a hazard whenever there is a substantial change in the estimate of the risks, in the personal or social acceptance of the risks, or in the plan of social management of the issue. The following cases illustrate.

Cyclamates. Until late 1969, cyclamates were used to sweeten everything from pickles to jellies to beverages (more than 5,600,000 pounds were put into 234,000,000 cases of soft drinks in 1965). They were deprived of their "generally recognized as safe" (GRAS) status and banned from foods by Herbert L. Ley, commissioner of the Food and Drug Administration, because of controversial new evidence that the compounds administered in massive doses to rats could induce bladder tumors—a risk not previously alleged. Cyclamates have been kept off the market ever since.[123]

DDT. Changes both in the public's values and in estimates of risk, influenced in large part by Rachel Carson's *Silent Spring*, led to the discrediting of this hitherto highly valued, widely used pesticide in the mid-1960s. The controversy was as much about the acceptability of the risks as it was about the magnitude and character of those risks.[124]

Mattresses. One of the first actions taken by the new Consumer Product Safety Commission was an attempt to manage the problem of bedroom fires by establishing strong standards for mattress flammability. Some consumers protested the price rise—"I don't even smoke, so why should I have to pay for an ignition-resistant mattress?"—and manufacturers asked for more time to develop the new mattresses. But in mid-1973 the commission ruled that all mattresses sold in the United States must pass specified cigarette-char tests.[125]

With cyclamates, strict regulatory interpretation of new scientific evidence raised the public issue; in short order cyclamates plummeted from "generally recognized as safe" to banishment. With DDT, a newly aroused public concern for the environment called for reassessment. With mattresses, governmental regulation based on performance standards was adopted to reduce the hazard.

---

[123]U. S. Congress, House of Representatives, Intergovernmental Relations Subcommittee of the Committee on Government Operations, *Hearing and Report on Regulation of Cyclamate Sweeteners* (1970); Robert B. Stenstrom, "Cyclamates," (report for the Program of Policy Studies in Science and Technology, George Washington University, April, 1971).

[124]See Chapter 6.

[125]Consumer Product Safety Commission, "Mattresses. Notice of amendments of flammability standard," *38 Federal Register,* 15095-15101 (June 8, 1973).

In each of the above cases a quiet, stable period was disrupted by a problem or crisis period marked by confusion and debate; eventually in each case resolution was reached—for the time being. Numerous similar cases come to mind: monosodium glutamate (MSG) and vinyl chloride echo the cyclamates problem; reform movements in coal mining and other hazardous occupations, reflecting changes in social values, resemble aspects of the DDT issue; mandatory automobile seat belts and childproof medicine bottle caps are reminiscent of the mattress flammability case.

For present purposes we will consider a "public problem" to be anything that looks like a public problem, whether that troubling appearance is justified rationally or not. No matter how accurate the perception of threat is, the public debate has to be resolved. Even if not of proper statistical, analytical notoriety, an electric appliance, doll, mascara, or pollutant that sufficiently outrages some public has to be attended to. The menace of hazards that are suspected but as yet unsubstantiated may be greatly feared, and sensational issues that seem minor by some criteria may command inordinate attention.

Safety problems often take on a complexion of crisis. The scenario is familiar. News of a newfound threat is broken by the media. Telephones start ringing. The accused offender mounts a hasty defense. Arguments rage not only over the risk itself but over who should bear the burden of proving the facts about the risk. Somebody eventually takes a suspending, conservative action. Then studies are undertaken, and relatively disinterested parties are consulted. Large amounts of money and attention are expended. Slowly, deep-seated economic and political forces take over, and the problem—as a public problem—is resolved. The true risk may or may not be reduced by all this; the alternatives that emerge may be even worse in some ways, or real improvement may have been achieved.

One thinks of the Great Cranberry Crisis of Thanksgiving, 1959: destruction of millions of pounds of cranberries that had become slightly contaminated by improper spraying with the weed killer, aminotriazole (ATZ); statements from the Food and Drug Administration about ATZ's carcinogenicity; politicians confidently eating cranberry sauce "just like the kind Mother used to make" on national television; the president of Ocean Spray Cranberries, Inc., telling the Secretary of Health, Education, and Welfare that "by one act disaster has come upon our industry. . . . By your statement you have placed the entire cranberry crop of the United States under suspicion, and we are confronted by a situation where we are adjudged guilty and must prove our innocence . . ."; the industry and government rushing to work out a plan to solve the problem; the President's Science Advisory Committee, personally instructed by the President to issue a report, invoking a "rule of reason" in interpreting the spirit of the Delaney principle; Congress, acting on the basis of a little-used 1935 law, voting ten million dollars in indemnification to the industry; and eventually, with simple changes in spraying practices and with an intensive publicity campaign, restoration of the cranberry to its former high public esteem.[126]

Elements of crisis can also be remembered in the brushed nylon "torch sweaters" problem of the 1950s, in which several women were badly burned simply by lighting cigarettes too near the fluffy, flammable sweaters. Then there was strontium-90 in milk, and mercury in swordfish, and steel-tipped children's darts. And the "Unsafe at Any Speed" Corvairs, and more recently, asbestos and the defoliant 2,4,5-T and vinyl chloride. . . .

Such issues pop up with so little warning and present so many nearly balanced but opposed arguments that public decisionmakers often make hasty decisions that must be reversed later. Examples easily come to mind. We find ourselves smiling with wry appreciation at science policy commentator Daniel Greenberg's "Dr. Grant Swinger's forecast for 1974" in which Dr. Swinger, "director of the Center for the Absorption of Federal Funds", predicted a January Food and Drug Administration ban on saccharin, with concomitant lifting of the ban on cyclamates; next a March removal of the ban on saccharin, with imposition of a ban on cyclamates; then in August, exoneration of cyclamates, with reimposition of the ban on saccharin. . . .[127] (At this writing, incidentally, saccharin, the principal artificial sweetener on the market, was newly under review by the Food and Drug Administration, and Abbott Laboratories was petitioning the Food and Drug Administration for reinstatement of its product sodium cyclamate.)[128]

No aspect of the national life escapes having crisis. We have mentioned three principal, and in a sense justifiable, causes of controversy over safety. It is not our task here to describe the occasional fumbling, venality, or wrangling over jurisdiction—the less justifiable causes of controversy—that afflict all major activities; those crises are not of a unique sort. What is special about safety crises is that they arise with little warning; their implications for well-being are taken personally and immediately by the affected public; the details of the technical assessments are often comprehensible only to a few specialists; and priorities are difficult to establish, because perceptions of the problems differ so much and because widely publicized immediate hazards distract attention from perhaps more important, but less visible, chronic ones.

[126]See Eugene Feingold, "The great cranberry crisis," in Edwin A. Bock, editor, *Government Regulation of Business: A Casebook* (Prentice-Hall, Englewood Cliffs, N. J., 1965) for a discussion of the episode as a regulatory issue.

[127]National Research Council, *Safety of saccharin and sodium saccharin in the human diet,* 1974.

[128]"Dr. Grant Swinger's forecast for 1974," *Science & Government Report IV,* no. 1 (January 1, 1974).

We often see specialists struggling to educate the lay public's sense of priorities. With air pollution, for example, health authorities urge reduction of the nitrogen oxides as well as the more readily perceived smoke, and the odorless pollutants as well as the smelly ones. This is a very modern phenomenon: we have so succeeded in controlling the great threats whose nature and magnitude made them un-ignorable (miserably hazardous workplaces, filthy drinking water, and a whole range of classical anemias and pestilences) that we are now free to worry about much less severe issues (noisy workplaces, side effects of fluoridating our drinking water, and bodily corpulence from overly rich diets). Most of the old menaces were only too obvious to everyone; now we depend on experts to sound the warnings. The question becomes, how do we know the experts are "right"? In view of the bitter opposition that arises from time to time, has the U. S. Public Health Service's endorsement and promotion of fluoridation been right? Those taking the alleged cancer cure "Krebiozen" believed that it was helping them and not hurting anybody else; in what sense was the government's decision to ban "Krebiozen" right? In a few pages we will return to the questions of government regulation and the uses of expert advice.

Finding ways to forestall crises is a perennial, but rarely realized, dream of administrators. The new Consumer Product Safety Commission has reasoned that it should survey accident patterns with some sophistication and establish its priorities on the basis of actual injury facts. As we will describe later, the commission conducts elaborate computer-assisted injury analyses and holds hearings on hazards that appear important. Of the thousands of classes of products over which it has jurisdiction, it has ranked the following as deserving the highest priority for accident-reduction attention: (1) bicycles; (2) stairs, ramps, and landings; (3) doors; (4) cleaning agents and caustic compounds; (5) tables; (6) beds; (7) football equipment and apparel; (8) swings, slides, seesaws, and playground climbing apparatus; (9) liquid fuels; and (10) architectural glass. That's just the top ten; hundreds more have been ranked. Both the desirability of constructing such a "most wanted" list, and the merits of particular rankings, have been subjects for heated debate. The commission hopes it can use the list to show that it is working on the hazards which are truly the most injurious to the American people, and conversely, that it can use the data to argue that certain sensational, crisis-inducing matters are really relatively minor.

WHO'S IN THE ARENA?

To call to mind just how big the safety arena can be, consider the problem of lead. The lead mining and processing industry supplies almost

3,000,000,000 pounds of lead a year in the United States alone. Manufacturers put it into storage batteries, fuel additives (more than 500,000,000
pounds were used in fuels in 1972), paints, ammunition, solder, and many
other products.[129] Lead in food is the responsibility of food processors and
the Food and Drug Administration. Lead in the atmosphere is principally
under the jurisdiction of the Environmental Protection Agency. Research
on health effects of lead, carried out in many different university, government, and industry laboratories, is supported by the Lead Industries
Association, the Environmental Protection Agency, the Public Health
Service, the American Petroleum Institute, and others. The World Health
Organization evaluates studies of health effects, as do committees of the
National Research Council. Occupational exposure is the concern of the
labor unions, the National Institute for Occupational Safety and Health
(NIOSH) of the Department of Health, Education and Welfare, and of the
Occupational Safety and Health Administration (OSHA) of the Department
of Labor; the AFL-CIO and OSHA have cooperatively established standards
for worker exposure. Special-interest groups such as the Urban Environment Coalition campaign for control of lead in the general environment.
Many government, industry, and academic groups work on the problem of
lead poisoning in children. Parents, tenants, and landlords work to settle
the lead paint issue. And the press carries accounts of this continuing debate.
For other major issues, the scene is just as complicated.[130]

And not only are there many people involved; the number of potential
hazards is simply staggering. A casual observer might think that DDT,
dieldrin, aldrin, and a few other compounds constitute the nation's pesticide
problem; actually, more than 35,000 different brand-name pesticide formu-
lations are registered currently with the Environmental Protection Agency.
One might think saccharin, and cyclamates, and a few dyes, thickeners, and
preservatives are our food additives problem; but 3600 are currently
approved by the Food and Drug Administration. More than 1500 compounds were listed recently by the Cosmetic, Toiletry and Fragrance
Association as being common ingredients in cosmetic preparations.[131] More
than 10,000 chemicals move in large volume in international commerce, and
tens of thousands more are used in lesser volume. The number of consumer

---

[129]Lead Industries Association, *U. S. Lead Industry Annual Review 1972.*

[130]For lists of the assignment of responsibilities for various hazards among the agencies of the government see Samuel S. Epstein and Richard D. Grundy, editors, *The Legislation of Product Safety* (MIT
Press, Cambridge, 1974).

[131]Cosmetic, Toiletry and Fragrance Association, Inc., *CFTA Cosmetic Ingredient Dictionary 1973.*

products on the market defies enumeration, and the items change constantly. Like counting the stars or anything else whose number and variety are incomprehensible, our inventorying could go on and on bemusedly, through household hazards, transportation hazards, and occupational hazards; but presumably the impression has been made. A lot of people are involved, and there are a lot of potential hazards.

Many of the people involved have technical backgrounds. Industrial research, design, development, testing, and engineering are done by technical people, many of whom move up through the corporate ranks to become top-level managers. Trade associations, such as the Pharmaceutical Manufacturers Association and the Crayon, Watercolor and Craft Institute, either have in their membership or retain technical experts. The National Safety Council, Consumers Union, the United Mine Workers, the AFL-CIO, the Union of Oil, Chemical, and Atomic Workers, and other private associations, testing laboratories, and labor unions all employ doctoral level scientists, health experts, and engineers to work on safety problems. So do insurance companies; a fire insuror without the capability to analyze the flammability potential of large, technically complicated structures would soon be out of business. The Environmental Defense Fund, the Health Research Group, and other public interest groups depend on both full-time and part-time technical advice. All the members of the scientific, medical, architectural, design, and engineering societies and academic faculties can influence the public's safety. A few members of the press have scientific training, as do some public officials. Many thousands of scientists serve the government as staff or advisors. The summary count would probably be surprisingly high.

A key conclusion from all this is that when one thinks of scientists and safety, one must think not only of the relative handful of safety professionals, such as safety engineers, or of the few eminent scientists appointed to high-level posts to review major issues, but beyond them and in many ways more importantly, of the far larger body of people implied by the above lists for whom safety is a partial but continuing responsibility.

Even though much of society's safety management rests with technically trained people, most of them have no special education or expertise in the concepts or practices of safety decisions per se. Worse, they may not even be sensitized to the problems. This may be one reason why we end up with foolishly designed, dangerous household goods and noisy, dirty environments, and why we are left feeling that many of those who are involved are not very good at it and that those who are not involved don't care about the issues. Many scientists do play responsible roles, of course, to which we now turn our attention.

MATTERS OF FACT, MATTERS OF VALUE

We have urged from the very beginning that the distinction between factual matters and value-laden ones be respected and identified openly. This even becomes an issue of responsibility; its implications will be important as we examine the roles technical people play.

One set of roles simply follows job titles: technical people work as researchers, designers, engineers, and so on, and an important fraction eventually moves into top-level administration and management.

A second set of roles, related to public decisionmaking, comprises (for want of better labels) assessors, advocates, and primary deciders. *Assessors* in principle try to maintain as much objectivity as possible, keeping their personal opinions in subjugation while they shape questions, grade the reliability of pieces of evidence, chart options, and plot the probable consequences of each of the options. It is a difficult stance, but with proper discipline and institutional arrangement it can be maintained. Scientists make assessments when they evaluate the environmental implications of several alternative plant sites for their industrial employer, or when they participate with a committee to review the impact of the Clean Air Act on national pulmonary health. The Congress's new Office of Technology Assessment is expected to work in this way as an institution.

Advocates are less strict about keeping their subjective convictions in check; they openly and vigorously champion particular courses of action. Technical people may lobby for the promotion or retardation of the nuclear power program, or they may urge their company management to expand production of a product they have personally been involved in developing.

Primary deciders work from some base of power. After listening to both assessors and advocates, they make decisions that cause action to be taken: a Food and Drug Administration commissioner makes a ruling on a drug, or a chief engineer approves the final design of a paper mill.

All of the above examples have implications for people's safety. Notice that institutions as well as by individuals can play these roles. Even though, obviously, the difference between assessing and advocating is just a matter of emphasis, that emphasis does vary over wide latitude.

Should scientists presume to judge for society what is safe? This question—part of the larger issue of the use of expertise—comes up perennially. One concern was expressed by Stanford geneticist Joshua Lederberg:

> Although valuable as a tool for solving the technological problems, expertise has distortions. . . . Besides the inherent problems of conflicts of interest and differing levels of competence, experts may also malfunction when they are asked, and fail to reject, the wrong *questions*. For example, a long series of

expert panels have reviewed the criteria for population exposure to environmental radiation from weapon-testing, medicine, and diverse peacetime nuclear power usages. The able, conscientious men on these panels (sometimes including the present author) had no difficulty in finding the common boundary of their knowledge of the hazards of a given dose of radiation. They could make rough estimates of the expected number of deaths and other miseries—but this was all they were competent to do. They should have refused to arrogate the wisdom—which they failed to do—to balance these costs against the anticipated benefits. Instead, the benefits were rarely analyzed, and when dealt with, were stated imprecisely. Indeed, what was demanded of such committees was a policy judgment, cloaked in technical detail.[132]

Similar indictments can be brought in many areas. But we should immediately point out that for scientists to default the appraisal of complex technological issues onto non-technically trained political leaders is not the solution. Hardly able to deal with the questions, or perhaps even to frame them properly, they would simply have to rely on their personal advisors—whose expertise and breadth would probably not equal that of such panels as the ones Dr. Lederberg refers to—or fall prey to the influence of strongly biased special interest lobbies. This is not to say that scientists should be left to take care of everything, an absurd notion. Nor is it to say that laymen should be wary of getting involved; on the contrary, what we so badly need is for laymen to press the science, to probe as incisively as possible, to define and debate the issues with sophistication.

In what we have referred to as the "any-man's-land", technical people are presumably as capable as others are, and in many cases more so, because of their breadth of experience and their habit of systematic thought. Not only can they understand the technical details and appreciate the nature of the uncertainties, but from experience they can often provide historical perspective on the problem, anticipate the public's acceptance of the risks fairly accurately, and think of alternatives and consequences that nontechnical people would miss.

Recognizing that they are making value judgments for the public, scientists can take several measures toward converting an "arrogation of wisdom" into a "stewardship of wisdom." First, they can leaven their discussions by including critical, articulate laymen in their group. Simply hearing or reading the opinions of a few laymen is hardly the same thing—and a courageous committee will confront itself with people who are not just token, well-meaning-but-fuzzy-brained "humanists", but with people

---

[132]Joshua Lederberg, "The freedom and the control of science: Notes from the ivory tower," *Southern California Law Review 45*, 609 (1972).

whose breadth and competence in an argument equals that of the rest of the group. Second, they can place on record their sources of bias and potential conflicts of interest, perhaps even stating their previous public positions on the issue. Third, they can identify the components of their decisions as being either scientific facts or matters of value judgment. Fourth, they can disclose in detail the specific bases upon which their assessments and appraisals are made. Fifth, they can reveal the degree of certainty with which the various parts of the decision are known. And sixth, they can express their findings in clear, jargon-free terms, in supplementary nontechnical presentations if not in the main report itself.

With any use of expertise a cluster of difficult questions comes up. Since the experts who know the most about a subject tend to have vested interests in it, how can conflicts of interest be avoided? Should advisors be made privy to the most confidential information but sworn to confidentiality—thereby ensuring a close working relationship and the best-informed advice—or should they be kept "outside" but left free, if conscience dictates, to disagree publicly with those they advise? Should advocates, or assessors, be consulted? Should the advisors be specialists in the field, or generalists chosen for their broader perspective and better balance—or would the inability of the latter to appreciate the technical details leave them poorly armed in debate? There are no universal answers. As they arise, public problems usually attract a diversity of experts, assessors *and* advocates, "inside" *and* "outside" commentators, specialists *and* generalists.[133]

Various institutional means have been proposed for preserving the distinction between knowledge and values and for managing hybrid problems. Most of them are based on adversary proceedings. Arthur Kantrowitz, chairman of Avco Everett Research Laboratory, Inc., has proposed an "institution for scientific judgment" which would "separate the scientific from the political and moral components of a mixed decision" and "separate judge from advocate."[134] Herbert L. Ley, former commissioner of the Food and Drug Administration, has proposed a "supreme court of food science" which would judge for the public what food additives are acceptable, what vitamins should remain unregulated, and what costs

[133]Robert Gilpin and Christopher Wright, *Scientists and National Policy-Making* (Columbia University Press, New York, 1964); general discussions of the roles of scientists in social decisionmaking appear in John M. Ziman, *Public Knowledge. An Essay Concerning the Social Dimension of Science* (Cambridge University Press, 1968); Victor C. Ferkiss, *Technological Man: The Myth and the Reality* (a Mentor book from New American Library, New York, 1969); Jerome R. Ravetz, *Scientific Knowledge and Its Social Problems* (Clarendon Press, Oxford, 1971); Joel Primack and Frank von Hippel, *Advice and Dissent. Scientists in the Political Arena* (Basic Books, New York, 1974).

[134]Arthur Kantrowitz, "Controlling technology democratically," *American Scientist 63*, 505-509 (1975).

should be paid for safe foods. Writing of the need for a new kind of agency to license pesticides and other widely dispersed chemicals, Harvard scholars Arthur J. Dyck and Herbert W. Richardson have said, "It is, perhaps, necessary to remind ourselves that there are no perfectly disinterested men and that the best way that such a public agency can function is by allowing all the special interests to plead their cases before a judicial board. Such a device is not foolproof, but is nevertheless needed to help to prevent use of environmental toxins in ways that would violate the principle of informed consent."[135] Few of these ideas have been tried; in a sense they are simply substitutes, not really different in kind, for exactly the tasks that elected and public officials are expected to carry out every day with their staffs and advisors.[136]

It is not yet clear whether such ideas will prove workable. Some precedent has been set by the Congress with its hearings on radiation, automobile safety and the seat belt issue, DDT, drug safety, air pollution, and cosmetics; but these hearings are rarely of a very critical nature. Several government agencies are currently instituting hearings procedures to develop matters of scientific fact. The Environmental Protection Agency is holding hearings on the pesticides dieldrin and aldrin and the defoliant 2,4,5-T; open petitions from all interested parties are entertained, then the administrative law judge who has heard the case submits his findings to the agency administrator for his consideration in passing a ruling. All petitions and arguments become a matter of public record. Similarly, the Consumer Product Safety Commission holds hearings "to get at the facts." Recently, for instance, in investigating why glass beverage containers had been so hazardous as to send 111,000 people to hospital emergency rooms in 1973, the commission heard the differing opinions and blameful accusations of bottle manufacturers, brewers, other beverage manufacturers, consumers, and consumer organizations.

The principal shortcoming of such hearings can be revealed simply by asking how "adversary" these "adversary proceedings" really are. Often they are just a series of testimonies read by experts who are never brought into direct confrontation with each other. Cross-examination is not usually allowed. Rather, direct battle over the facts, if it occurs at all, takes place as

---

[135]Arthur J. Dyck and Herbert W. Richardson, "The moral justification for research using human subjects," National Academy of Sciences/National Research Council, *Use of Human Subjects in Safety Evaluation of Food Chemicals,* 240 (1967).

[136]For further discussion see Allen Mazur, "Disputes between experts," *Minerva 11,* 243-262 (1973); Louis H. Mayo, "Scientific method, adversarial system, and technology assessment," Monograph Number 5, The George Washington University Program of Policy Studies in Science and Technology, National Technical Information Service PB 196 638 (1970).

a free-for-all in the mass media. The well meant but ineffectual hearings simply provide a forum for opening reports that escalate into exchanges of biased statistics, political flanking maneuvers, and attacks on person—all distorted further by shallow, sensational media coverage. As a result, the hearings are left with an archival record of unexamined and perhaps biased and unreliable science, while the newspapers publish a limited, oversimplified and perhaps sensationalized account of the challenge and counter-challenge of ideas that more truly characterize the scientific process.

We should expect adversary proceedings that are *really* adversary to be extremely useful. In discussing Alvin Weinberg's description of "trans-scientific problems," Harvey Brooks has summarized:

> Adversary procedures may be especially valuable in bringing out unanalyzed evaluative assumptions or premises which underlie the testimony of experts when they deal with trans-scientific issues. Adversary procedures are also important in circumstances when greater and greater economic, political or professional commitments have been made to a particular line of action, and when such commitments are to be either greatly scaled up or down as a result of a policy decision based on scientific and trans-scientific testimony.[137]

We close this section with the following provocative statement from Eugene Rabinowitch, the biophysicist who from the end of the Manhattan Project until his recent death dealt with these difficult issues as editor of the *Bulletin of the Atomic Scientists*:

> In adversary proceedings in which science or one of its applications (such as technology, medicine or psychiatry) are involved, both sides enlist the cooperation of experts—scientists for the prosecution and scientists for the defense, scientists for the government and scientists for the opposition. This procedure makes a mockery of science; in fact, it often comes dangerously close to its prostitution.
>
> Juries, parliaments and electorates, when called upon to judge between con-testing claims, often are unable to judge the arguments of their scientific experts rationally, and often rely on the impression the competing experts make on them, on their formal credentials, and on the forensic quality and vigor of their presentation.
>
> In the controversy over nuclear bomb tests, some scientists, called upon by opponents of testing, emphasized the absolute number of radiation-induced bone cancers and leukemias likely to be caused by continued testing in the atmosphere; while other scientists, called upon by advocates of testing, stressed the low number of expected victims, compared to the general incidence of these

---

[137]Harvey Brooks, "Science and trans-science," *Minerva 10*, 484-486 (1972).

malignancies. The first group of scientists used the data to claim that continued testing in the atmosphere would be criminal, while the second group used the data to argue that there is no reason to discontinue the tests. Laymen, including legislators, concluded that one cannot trust scientists: some of them say, 'Stop tests—they are too dangerous'; others, 'Go on, you will not notice the difference.' Yet, as scientists, the adversary experts did not disagree on the facts of the situation; they disagreed only on moral conclusions which they derived from these facts—a disagreement in which the judgment of scientists is no more, while no less, valid than that of any other citizen *cognizant of the facts*.

Scientific experts called upon in litigation or in political controversies should not be used as partisan assistants in the adversary process, but as impartial investigators to provide an agreed upon summary of the relevant facts as well as the logical derivations from these facts. If needed, the summary should clearly present differing interpretations of the scientific evidence and differing moral or political presumptions leading to different practical conclusions. ...

Scientists, psychiatists, physicians and technologists should be asked to analyze a problem, and to render their conclusions, without advance presumption as to what point of view they are to defend. If, at a certain point, their conclusions begin to be affected by extra-scientific reasons, they must have sufficient intellectual honesty to state: 'Up to this point, I spoke as a scientist; from here on I will speak also as a politically, ethically or ideologically committed citizen. ...'

Scientists will not always be able to make this distinction clearly; but, at least society must not encourage them to behave unscientifically, to conceal their bias, or to resort to untruth or suppression of a part of evidence.[138]

The pressure of the issues in this time of "future shock" means that we had better learn to manage these issues, or else.

IN THE PUBLIC INTEREST

The public interest movement begun in the last decade is with us to stay. Many of the movement's most visible accomplishments have concerned safety: of automobiles, of pesticides, of food additives. Perpetuation of the spirit of that movement is assured not only by the existence of many active organizations and competent individuals, but also by the general change in the national attitude as reflected in new laws, such as the Freedom of Information Act (Public Law PL 90-23) and the Federal Advisory Committee Act (Public Law 92-463), which enlarge the public's access to government deliberations. Public advocacy has gained a new responsibility.

---

[138]Eugene Rabinowitch, "Back into the Bottle?" *Science and Public Affairs*, 19-23 (April, 1973).

An offshoot activity, sometimes referred to as "public interest science", has arisen because of what is seen as "the growing public awareness of the dangerous consequences of leaving the exploitation of technology under the effective control of special industrial and governmental interests." Its strategy is "taking the issue to the public." Enormous persistence and skill are required, as well as a good and timely case, to be heard above the din that accompanies everyday living in this country."[139]

The tactics employed—elaborate legal action, massive public appeals, and work by large coalitions of special groups—have not been so extensively used before in dealing with technological public issues. There is little doubt about the effectiveness of some of the campaigns for control of pesticides, abatement of noise, less adulteration of food, less risky cosmetics, and stricter management of the nuclear power industry.[140]

What has to be questioned now is how effective and responsible the public interest organizations will prove to be in the long run. They are largely self-appointed advocates, not truly public representatives, and are not under formal guidance from the public. After sensational, crusading beginnings focused on immediate, visible issues, will they be able to maintain tough internal quality control as they grow? So far, the most effective campaigns have been centered upon a few highly talented individuals; how will large organizations evade the hobbles of Parkinson's law and its corollaries? Will they learn to set priorities reasonably, taking on important tasks? Will they find ways of tackling problems and gaining support without having to resort to instigating crises? Will their activities unnecessarily raise society's costs? Most importantly, will they be able to avoid developing such strong biases and vested interests that they become just like all the other special interest lobbies? The movement has reached the age for evaluation.

In passing we should note that even the "openness" movement, purely motivated though it may be, is turning out to have drawbacks as well as

---

[139]Frank von Hippel and Joel Primack, "Public interest science," *Science 177*, 1166-1171 (1972).

[140]Theodore Berland, *The Fight for Quiet* (Prentice-Hall, Englewood Cliffs, New Jersey, 1970); James Turner, *The Chemical Feast: Report on the Food and Drug Administration* (Grossman, New York, 1970); Rosemary Chalk, "Citizen Participation in Technical Planning," *Public Science Newsletter 4*, No. 6, 4-11 (1973); Steven Ebbin and Raphael Kasper, *Citizen Groups and the Nuclear Power Controversy* (MIT Press, Cambridge, 1974); Priscilla W. Laws, *Medical and Dental X-Rays: A Consumer's Guide to Avoiding Unnecessary Radiation Exposure* (Health Research Group, 2000 P Street, N.W., Washington, D.C. 20036, 1974); Minnesota Public Interest Research Group, *Cosmetics and the Cosmetic Industry, or, "The Great Cover Up,"* (MPIRG, 3036 University Avenue Southeast, Minneapolis, Minnesota, 1973; reprinted in U. S. Senate Committee on Labor and Public Welfare, *Hearings on the Cosmetic Safety Act of 1974* (February 21-22, 1974); Joel Primack and Frank von Hippel, *Advice and Dissent. Scientists in the Political Arena* (Basic Books, Inc., New York, 1974).

accomplishments. It does provide leverage allowing citizens access to meetings and documents, but at the same time it tends to force many decisions
further into the bureaucratic matrix. Decisions that once were made around
a table and confirmed by letter are now made over the telephone; decisions
that once were made in announced but confidential conferences are now
made in "executive committee" rump sessions following duly conducted
public meetings. And, in avoidance of red tape, decisions are now often
made by administrators without consulting *any* outside advisors. Again,
evaluation is called for to examine whether we are achieving not only the
statutory requirements of the public access acts but also the spirit and intent
of those acts.

IN THE COURTS

The courts can be thought of as being a forum for reappraising the
worth of actions, relative to society's evolving collective moral convictions.
By hearing charges of misrepresentation, mislabelling, negligence, and
fraud, by resolving jurisdictional disputes among regulatory agencies, and
by guiding the execution of public laws, the courts continually recalibrate
the yardstick of social values.

In recent years the courts have been noticeably more active in the areas
of environmental, occupational, and product safety. The prospect of
financial penalty and adverse publicity from lawsuits has become an important deterrent to rash action.

There has come to be increasing intercourse in the United States between
the legal system and the technical community. Some of the interaction is on
a personal level, as a recent review describes:

> The technical community today faces a serious challenge in the legal arena of
> product liability litigation. Hundreds of thousands of product liability cases
> are filed each year, each requiring technical expertise of varying degrees of
> complexity. Scientists and engineers are called upon to evaluate diverse products
> involved with injuries and to communicate their findings in an environment
> that often appears foreign to their own technical problem-solving processes.

That review cited John W. Wade's list of seven criteria governing litigation over the reasonableness of a hazard:

    (i) the usefulness and desirability of the product;

    (ii) the availability of other and safer products to meet the same need;

    (iii) the likelihood of injury and its probable seriousness;

116

(iv) the obviousness of the danger;

(v) common knowledge and normal public expectation of the danger (particularly for established products);

(vi) the avoidability of injury by care in use of the product (including the effect of instructions or warnings); and

(vii) the ability to eliminate the danger without seriously impairing the usefulness of the product or making it unduly expensive.

Technically trained people are often called upon to sort through these criteria, identify those which are amenable to technical analysis, and then deliver such analyses in expert testimony. The authors of the above review recommend a "seriated" trial format in which, insofar as possible, "questions related to product integrity and technical causation are treated apart from the other issues of liability."[141]

In some cases the involvement of the technical community in safety proceedings is more collective. For instance, volunteer standards-setting organizations are finding their status changing as questions like the following arise: "If a large building is destroyed by a fire whose fury is intensified by high temperature decomposition of standard quality polyurethane foam insulation, who should be found at fault—the insulation manufacturer, the builder, or the trade or government organization that certified the insulation as safe?" If such a case should come to trial, the pivotal issue of whether the insulation did substantially feed the fire would have to be settled on the basis of testimony by technical experts. And the standards organization might well find itself in court.

The questions of who should bear the costs of safety, and where the courts should assign those costs, is under continuing debate. A prominent view of product safety is that propounded by the National Commission on Product Safety. The Commission supported the common-law mechanism of compensation. It argued for the doctrine of strict liability, under which the consumer need only prove that he was injured by a product that was in some sense defective and unreasonably hazardous. It argued that the quality of warnings should be considered in decisions on defectiveness; that certifying organizations be held liable ("truth-in-certification"); that the Uniform Commercial Code be changed to make suing for breach of warranty easier; and that small claims provisions be expanded.[142]

---

[141]Henry R. Piehler, Aaron D. Twerski, Alvin S. Weinstein, and William A. Donaher, "Product liability and the technical expert," *Science 186*, 1089-1093 (1974); J. W. Wade, "Strict tort liability of manufacturers," *Southwest Law Journal 19*, 5-25 (1965).

[142]National Commission on Product Safety, *Final Report* (1970).

Similar considerations obtain in environmental and occupational problems. Each of these points has been fought over in many forums, as have such important companion issues as class actions and the assignment of burden of proof. The courts are conservative, in that they make their decisions on the basis of precedent; they tend to reflect, rather than initiate, social change (although certainly they do catalyze much widespread change). They usually act only *after* people have actually been injured. And they are slow, legendarily slow, and costly both to the litigants and to society as a whole.

IN THE MEDIA

The public's understanding of safety problems and the intensity of its concern over them are strongly influenced by the news media. Quite often, as we have seen, a crisis breaks out with little warning, sending the press corps scrambling not only for the facts but for interpretation ("But Doctor, what *is* mesothelioma ...?"). From time to time reporters accuse scientists of speaking obliquely or suppressing information, while technical people scornfully accuse the press of a kind of sensational muckraking that passed its peak of usefulness sixty years ago.

Among scientists, fear of being misconstrued is strong, and justifiably. Hysterical public reactions do not help the cause of rationality. Frequently, a laboratory comes upon some evidence which casts doubt on the safety of something—tenuous, uncertain evidence, perhaps, which will need to be strengthened over the coming months. Conscience dictates that the news should be announced, both to warn those who are at risk and who may wish to exercise caution, and to alert other researchers who may be on the track of the same problem. What is needed is a cautious, carefully qualified, responsible public statement. Sometimes this is achieved; sometimes not. When it is not, irremediable social damage may be done.

In one sense it is inevitable that the general media presentation of safety issues will be skewed, in that sensational events will always get disproportionate coverage; they do make "stories," after all, whereas the continuing glacial menaces to which we are subjected make hot copy only when a crisis breaks out or when an unusually enterprising investigative reporter writes a critical story.

In this and other areas the media need to develop better continuing relations with the technical community, if for no other reason than to get interpretive help. As always, the media cannot too strongly be encouraged to do their own investigating instead of simply reworking press releases; to resist being "used" by special interest factions; to follow up preliminary breaking stories with better balanced in-depth reports; and to strive in their reporting to make forcible distinctions between issues of value judgment and empirical, factual ones.

ON BEING, AND BEING HELD, RESPONSIBLE

Anyone who has read to this point has surely become so concerned about issues of responsibility that further introduction to this section is unnecessary. Every sector of society has its ethical problems. We will focus on those concerning scientists and other technical people, for the most part limiting ourselves to those concerning issues of personal safety.

In essence, the issue is posed by the following questions. Should technically trained people be expected to bear any social responsibilities different from those borne by others? Why? What are the unique obligations? And further, can all the obligations be met simply by individuals working alone, or are there in addition some responsibilities requiring technical people to act collectively?

Most discussions of these questions are not very useful: either they harangue the reader about how technology has sent the world to the brink of oblivion, without admitting to their scapegoating or suggesting a way back from the brink; or else they preach a benign sermon reducing ethics to moral goodness, and merely plead with people to be virtuous. We will try to avoid these extremes. Our approach will be to describe briefly what society's expectations are, show that they form a general pattern of obligations that both scientists and nonscientists recognize and that scientists seem to accept in principle, point out that this responsibility is based on a tacit but real compact between the technical professions and society, and argue that this compact is fairly workable as long as it is enforced and renegotiated to keep up with the needs of the times.

The public does have special expectations of technical people. "I don't know anything about building materials, but I would certainly expect anyone who designs a hospital, nursing home, or school to make it fireproof." "If scientists learn that a food additive or drug is harmful, it is unethical for them not to warn the public." "It is wrong for a research chemist or engineer to develop a manufacturing process that will expose workers to conditions that, for health reasons, the researcher himself wouldn't tolerate." "A designer or engineer who designs or approves a dangerous toy or appliance should be drummed out of the profession." Such opinions are widespread among both technical and nontechnical people. They fall into several different categories, as we will show.

119

[Since this book has emphasized that value judgments should be labelled as such, the author feels bound to state that the following is strictly his personal opinion; nonetheless, he believes that it is widely shared.]

Scientists, engineers, designers, architects, physicians, public health experts, and other technically trained people *do* have special responsibilities to the rest of society with respect to personal safety. Some principal kinds of risks which ought to be taken upon the conscience of the technical community are:

1. Technically complex risks whose intricacies are comprehensible only to highly trained people;

2. Risks that can be significantly reduced by applying new technology or by improving the application of existing technology;

3. Risks constituting public problems whose technical components need to be distinguished explicitly from their social and political components so that responsibilities are assigned properly;

4. Technological intrusions on personal freedom made in the pursuit of safety; and

5. Risks whose possible consequences appear so grave or irreversible that prudence dictates the urging of extreme caution, even before the risks are known precisely.

Notice that we have said that these problems *should be taken as matters of conscience* by the technical community. Whether the verb describing the action should be *protecting,* or *watching over,* or *looking out for,* or *issuing a warning,* depends on the situation. The specific response might be doing an experiment, raising an issue before a professional society, blowing the whistle on an employer, exerting political leverage, or aiding a legislator or administrator in untangling the parts of a public issue. We will mention some examples of the above categories; a single problem often belongs to several of them.

1. *Technically complex risks whose intricacies are comprehensible only to highly trained people.* The complexities of deciding whether chemicals are carcinogenic, or of evaluating the design of such large structures as bridges, dams, tunnels, and aircraft, obviously leave such problems squarely in the province of those with advanced training and experience. And this goes beyond "You made it; you worry about it"; technical people must also be relied upon to predict the consequences of natural disasters and other such hazards.

120

2. *Risks that can be significantly reduced by applying new technology or by improving the application of existing technology.* Here we think of aircraft landing guidance systems, tidal wave warning devices, vaccines against disease, and occupational protective measures. In most cases only technical people can envision the possibilities.

3. *Risks constituting public problems whose technical components need to be distinguished explicitly from their social and political components so that responsibilities are assigned properly.* Scientists need to point out over and over that although developing nuclear power is a technical matter, as is the development of solar power, deciding how much of what kind of commitment to make to each of the two programs is a thoroughly hybrid scientific-political issue. They then need to stay involved as the tasks are "factored apart"; otherwise, politicians may overlook some issues that are obvious only to science, or scientists may find themselves having to make social decisions under illegitimate pretenses.

4. *Technological intrusions on personal freedom made in the pursuit of safety.* This category includes the responsibility of researchers to protect their experimental subjects, with respect not only to their physical health but to their emotional well-being and personal liberty as well. It might conceivably also include warning of some of the subtle intrusions on freedom implied by certain government decisions, such as requirements that all school children submit to genetic screening.

5. *Risks whose possible consequences appear so grave or irreverisble that prudence dictates the urging of extreme caution, even before the risks are known precisely.* Wearing the prophet's cape is itself a risky business. Unless it is done with care, not only is the specific prophecy ignored, but the prophet loses his credibility. Nevertheless, scientists are counted upon to issue warnings about especially insidious hazards, to prescribe safeguards, and to raise public awareness of the danger. Some scientists are now doing this with radioactive waste problems—particularly with the toxic and exceedingly long-lived material, plutonium—and with the upper-atmospheric ozone problem. In the latter case, for instance, even if the effects of freons, SST exhausts, and so forth eventually turn out not to be serious threats (it is too early to tell), it will not have been wrong to investigate—indeed, because of the extraordinary potential gravity of the risks it would be irresponsible *not* to see that they get appraised.

These are but a few of the social responsibilities of scientists, but they are among the most readily identified and agreed upon. There are others: obligations to frame risk and safety issues in proper relation to factors of equity, cost, efficacy, and so on, and obligations to interpret new findings for the lay public. There are also attitudinal and procedural responsibilities such as defending against suppression, misinterpretation, and falsification of data, and preserving the distinction between factual and valuational decisions. In all of these tasks nonscientists can be enlisted for reinforcement. But scientists must often be depended upon to take the initiative.

These responsibilities have several deep origins. Basically they arise, in congruence with all major moral philosophies, from the conviction that every person has a general responsibility for the well-being of his fellow men. Reflecting this, the common law has held through the centuries that anyone who becomes aware of the possibility of danger has a responsibility to warn those at risk. But we are obliged to push further and ask whether, in this age of cultural specialization, there isn't more to the issue—for if we don't press, we may be left simply making vague exhortations to virtue.

When we examine what society expects, we find that it does look to the technical community for warning, guidance, and protection, in the kinds of situations we have described and in others as well. Highly trained people are definitely seen as having special status. Given this, a key to developing a compelling ethical argument, and to understanding why the lay public feels as it does, seems to reside in the notion of professionalism.

Over the years a tacit but nonetheless real compact has developed. Society *invests in* the training and professional development of scientists and other technical people. It invests heavily; substantial public subsidy of one form or another goes to virtually every college, university, medical school, field station, and research facility in the United States. By and large the professions are left free to govern themselves, control admission to membership, choose their direction of research, enforce the quality of work, and direct the allocation of public funds within their subject area.

Concomitantly, society *invests with* the professions and their institutions certain trusts, among them a trust that the professions will watch over the well-being of society, including its safety. As Berkeley sociologist William Kornhauser has expressed it, "Professional responsibility is based on the belief that the power conferred by expertise entails a fiduciary relationship to society."[143]

---

[143]William Kornhauser, *Scientists in Industry*, 1 (University of California Press, Berkeley, 1962).

This "fiduciary relationship," or what we have called a tacit compact, is what gives rise to the ethical "oughts."

Within this compact, the professions develop two kinds of obligations. The first is an ethics governing maintenance of the profession; it consists of a set of restraints mutually agreed to by peers, and it shades into being an etiquette. The second is a commitment to the service of society as well as to individual clients. This commitment usually grows slowly. By stepping into gaps during crises, or by deliberately staking out pieces of social territory, the profession comes to be responsible for special matters. For example, geneticists have not only dispassionately studied our chromosomes as objects of scientific curiosity, but, slowly and by subtle stages, they have come to be guardians of this genetic treasure as well. In part, this guardianship is self-appointed. It is appreciated and it is rarely contested. Because this particular compact seems to work—that is, geneticists get their support and freedom, and society gets protection for its genes—society now *expects* geneticists, as a matter of their ethical responsibility, to continue their watch for mutagenic menaces. And in general geneticists seem to accept the responsibility. Similar expectations are held in many areas. The obligations go far beyond the duties for which people draw their salaries, and the seriousness of some of the possible errors of omission exceeds anything people can be held legally liable for.

From time to time, the compact is modified. Someone, perhaps an outsider, perhaps a member of the profession, levels a charge of irresponsibility or corruption. In response, the profession purges itself of charlatans or revises its code of practice, or the public withdraws its support or stiffens its licensing requirements for admission to the profession. Such "clean house, or else we'll clean it for you" challenges are currently being laid, for instance, against researchers who are thought to be taking unethical advantage of research subjects and against industrial scientists who have allegedly suppressed data about carcinogens in their factories.

The professions not only face inward and enforce their codes, but they also face outward to support and defend members who meet resistance in discharging their obligations. On occasion, an employer may interpret a professional's act of conscience as an act of disloyalty or worse, and harass him or threaten to fire or sue. The principal recourse for the repressed professional may be to retreat to the sanctuary of the guildhall (the metaphor is apt; the high guilds, such as the goldsmiths', set an effective and honorable precedent). In several recent instances, professional societies have provided legal defense and supportive publicity for members

123

who were suffering unduly for "blowing the whistle" on what they believed were unconscionable situations.[144] Many professional societies now have ethics committees to review these matters in general and to prepare for contingencies. A society may choose not to defend its members' particular stands, but rather to defend their right to issue warnings and take stands without recrimination. A society may be able to advise its members on the most reasonable ways to exert influence. And a society may take the lead in converting an accusatory confrontation into a more broadly based assessment.

As this century has careened along it has brought an increasing need for a collective shouldering of responsibility. The one-to-one personal relationships that once governed ethical conduct have been supplanted by more diffuse ones involving many intermediaries. Industrial scientists plan their research by committee. Engineers who design tunnels and dams interact with their ultimate public clients only indirectly, through managers, attorneys, and the officials who supervise public contracts. Physicians may still carry the wand of Aesculapius, but they do so in the context of one of the nation's largest businesses. Two sorts of diffuseness enlarge the collective dimension. First, the cliency is expanding, often in the interest of social justice: a national health care system that intends to reach every citizen has quite different ethical dimensions from a free-market private physician system. And second, as we confront hazards that are more diffuse, we often realize that *nobody* has considered that the problem was specifically his concern: there is no International Agency for the Supervision of the Ozone Layer.

We try to manage these problems by government action, building in mechanisms of accountability where possible; and we test the justice of specific actions in the courts, as when people feel that they are being unfairly denied medical care. Beyond that, and usually leading it, we have to depend on action by communities of scholars and coteries of professionals—hence the obligations we listed earlier.

Two current cases exemplify some of the difficulties. Three engineers in California, backed to a limited extent by several engineering societies, have pressed suit against the Bay Area Rapid Transit (BART) system for firing them after they publicly protested that the automatic train control systems their companies were developing for BART were inadequate and not up to the best professional standards with regard to passenger safety.

---

[144]Ralph Nader *et al.*, editors, *Whistle Blowing: The Report of the Conference on Professional Responsibility* (Bantam, New York, 1971).

The dispute raises complex questions about how great the risks really were, whether they should have been considered acceptable, how engineers should play their roles, how corporations should handle dissension, and what the professional societies should do.[145] In another case, an international group of biologists has voluntarily convened itself to discuss whether and how to control certain genetics experiments that would have bizarre, disastrous consequences if they ran amok.[146]

There is little precedent for either case, so it is not surprising that neither has been handled with assurance. In the BART case, the engineering societies were not well prepared to act and could muster only limited support. Perhaps for lack of experience and guidance, the three engineers party to the suit were not able to pursue the case through the courts to completion; the case has reportedly had to be settled out of court, thus setting only weak legal precedent. In the genetic experiments case, the scientists involved continue to suffer the anguish of not even being able to reach a firm consensus on the issue, and they are hard pressed to take any action other than to issue stern pronouncements, plead for prudence, and cross their collective fingers that researchers will be careful.

We have developed the above arguments because we believe they are important. They are by no means the sole guide to action. There can be no substitute for honesty, courage, sacrifice, and the other manifestations of high morality. Nor should legal and other sanctions fail to be applied: enforcible building codes can be adopted to supplement voluntary action; duties can be made a matter of contractual responsibility; and falsification of records is cause for lawsuit. There are many obligations in addition to ethical ones. The ethical ones are of a special sort, though, and urgently deserve to be developed.

The great questions of responsibility will remain with us. Is simply providing information or issuing warnings a sufficient response, or ought those with the knowledge do more? How is responsibility passed up through administrative and managerial hierarchies? In what sense is tacit acquiescence in a misleading scheme irresponsible (as when corporate scientists who know better say nothing when their company makes false

[145]Gordon D. Friedlander, *IEEE Spectrum 11*, 69-76 (October, 1974); Gordon D. Friedlander, "Fixing BART," *IEEE Spectrum 12*, 43-45 (February, 1975).

[146]Nicholas Wade, "Genetics: Conference sets strict controls to replace moratorium," *Science 187*, 931-935 (1975); Stuart Auerbach, "And man created risks," *Washington Post* (March 9, 1975).

claims for its products or evades pollution control laws)? To what extent should those who generate scientific and technological innovations be responsible for their subsequent application?[147]

---

[147]General discussion of the ethical responsibilities of technical people may be found in the following sources: Warren O. Hagstrom, *The Scientific Community* (Basic Books, New York, 1965); Don K. Price, *The Scientific Estate* (Harvard University Press, Cambridge, Mass., 1965); William Kornhauser, *Scientists in Industry* (University of California, Berkeley, 1962); Jerome R. Ravetz, *Scientific Knowledge and Its Social Problems* (Oxford University Press, London, 1971); Philip Siekevitz, editor, "The social responsibility of scientists," *Annals of the New York Academy of Sciences 196,* article 4 (1972); "Science and its public: The changing relationship," *Daedelus 103* (Summer, 1974); Joel Feinberg, *Doing and Deserving: Essays in the Theory of Responsibility* (Princeton University Press, 1974); National Academy of Sciences/Institute of Medicine, *Ethics of Health Care* (1974); Joel Primack and Frank vo n Hippel, *Advice and Dissent. Scientists in the Political Arena* (Basic Books, New York, 1974); John T. Edsall, "Scientific freedom and responsibility," Report of the American Association for the Advancement of Science, Committee on Scientific Freedom and Responsibility, *Science 188,* 687-693 (1975).

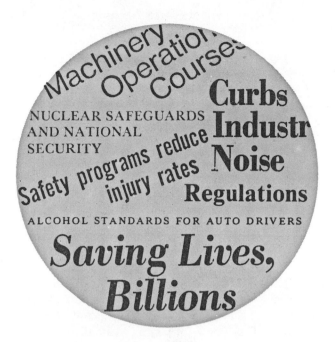

Machinery Operation Courses

NUCLEAR SAFEGUARDS AND NATIONAL SECURITY

Curbs Industr

Safety programs reduce injury rates

Noise Regulations

ALCOHOL STANDARDS FOR AUTO DRIVERS

Saving Lives, Billions

5

Making Safe

The actions that can be taken to safeguard the public include such varied approaches as regulatory control, registration, and licensing; special product design; application of standards; education of consumers and workers; and monitoring and maintaining surveillance.

Strategies for protection can be aimed at any of three principal factors: the exposure hazard itself (defective products, contaminants in the environment), victim error (user ignorance, carelessness), and what might be called aggravating circumstances. Preventive actions may be taken, as by designing safety features in products, educating product users, and setting emission standards for pollutants. Or after-the-fact remedial and compensatory measures may be taken, as by awarding legal damages for injury. The timing and selection of safeguarding actions depends on whether the hazard is regarded as safe until proven unsafe, or whether it is mistrusted as unsafe until proven safe. Some safeguarding responsibilities are assumed solely by individuals, and others are entrusted to the government or other social institutions.

MAKING SAFE THROUGH REGULATION

With the growth in scale and centralization of our society—from the early days of exploding steamship boilers and collapsing coal mines, to the first colliding gasoline buggies, through the turn-of-the-century threats mentioned in our introductory chapter, to medical X-rays, and continuing through the present—we have increasingly relied upon government regulation to manage our hazards.[148] The Environmental Protection Agency registers pesticides. The Food and Drug Administration licenses antibiotics. The states license drivers. The Consumer Product Safety Commission requires that certain household chemicals be provided with warning labels or special packaging. The Occupational Safety and Health Administration establishes workplace standards. The Federal Trade Commission enforces product warranties. Cities inspect meat.

To the perennial question, "Under what conditions does the government step in and regulate?" we would answer, without meaning to be cynical, that the government regulates whenever public pressure builds up to make it regulate. Consumer outrage about drugs leads to new legislation, perhaps amendment of the food and drug laws. Pressure from medical experts, public interest groups, and labor unions leads to regulation of an occupational hazard. The process is no more arcane—or systematic—than that. There is no single set of general criteria by which the government decides whether to take regulatory action. In general, the government tends to regulate in order to protect the people from those things against which they are unable to protect themselves. Regulation is widely applied to problems, such as environmental pollution, in which actions taken by an individual may affect many other people who are not directly able to control the offender's actions. Regulation is used to protect the especially vulnerable, as when strict fire codes are

---

[148]For historical perspective, see "Health and safety laws," *Encyclopedia Brittanica.*

established for nursing homes. The government also tends to intervene when, as with highly technological products such as pharmaceuticals, pesticides, and food additives, appraising and controlling the issue requires a technical expertise few people possess.

Theorists usually say that regulatory intervention by the government is required when ordinary market mechanisms fail—when, in a given situation, net costs to society are greater than net private costs. The question, however, is what "fail" means. There is little disagreement that free-enterprise market pressures alone fail to control such highly technological hazards and general environmental problems as those referred to above. And short of an unenvisionable revolution in driver attitudes, the highways would be even more hazardous if their use were not heavily regulated.

But consider the seemingly simple product, the ladder. Hearings on the safety of ladders brought testimony that "cheaper ladders are less well constructed and have few if any of the better safety features," lacking nonslip feet and step treads, having "too many sharp corners, rough edges and places where hands could be caught," and being "difficult to handle for erecting and carrying." Summarizing its findings, the National Commission on Product Safety concluded that

> The household ladder is not likely to be used in a consistently prudent manner ... While consumers are presumably aware of the risk of injury in using a ladder, seemingly they do not realize how often certain common practices (twisting the ladder more than it can tolerate, or standing on the top step) create danger ... We asked why the industry does not modify designs since the common household ladder is a hazard even when it meets existing standards. The answer according to them is that, given a choice of several ladder styles and prices, including those built for household use, it is unlikely that the consumer will be willing to pay for the safety factors. Unless safety features are mandatory, the buyer commonly opts for a slight saving in price.[149]

From the Commission's point of view, market mechanisms have failed to make ladders safe. So the question becomes, should the government make safety features mandatory? "I've never fallen off a ladder, and besides, I only use one once a year to clean my gutters; why shouldn't I be free to buy any kind of ladder I want?" A response might be, "But you probably

---

[149]National Commission on Product Safety, *Final Report*, 25-26 (1970).

don't know just how dangerous ladders really are." Which would bring a rejoinder something like, "Sure I do; and I don't mind taking that risk. I'm careful ..."

It is difficult to generalize on attitudes. A person who expects the Food and Drug Administration to use its expertise and power to "keep those additives out of my food" may at the same time be outraged that the agency is considering controlling the formulation of vitamins. A single individual may insist that traffic lights be installed, complain about enforcement of speed limits, be unenthusiastic but tolerant about seatbelts, and firmly oppose making motorcycle helmets mandatory.

Describing hazards in terms of the array of considerations laid out in Chapter 3 can be useful in analyzing trends. Voluntariness of exposure and the availability of alternatives are obviously important criteria in the examples given in the preceding paragraph. Things such as glass doors that are quite likely to be involved in hazardous misuse may warrant regulatory supervision, such as requiring shatterproof glass or highly visible warning markers.

The demand for regulation—for a Consumer Product Safety Commission that bans 677 kinds of toys in two years—seems to be a crying out at the futility of dealing with the multiplicity of hazards confronting us these days.[150] People call for regulation almost reflexively, as though it were either a panacea or the last resort. A 1974 Harris poll of the public's views about the safety of consumer products revealed that "home pesticides, room heaters, automobiles, and power lawn mowers top the list of products causing greatest public concern. ... The public is not only worried about product safety but also feels that the federal government is not doing a highly effective job of enforcing safety standards." Tighter regulation was viewed as a solution to the problem: "Seventy-seven per cent of the buying public favor 'the federal government developing more extensive standards for product safety'."[151] But it is not clear whether the poll would have brought the same reponse if all the costs and encroachments on purchasing freedom had been fully understood.

It is not our purpose here to discuss the general issue of government regulation, which is complicated by considerations of feasibility, cost distribution, justice, and "Big Brotherism"; those issues are not unique to safety matters.[152] More and more the question is being raised, are we

[150]Consumer Product Safety Commission, "Banned products list," volume III, part 1, special holiday issue (October 1, 1974).

[151]Louis Harris, "Product safety: Stricter federal controls sought," Washington Post (July 15, 1974).

[152]Peter H. Schuck, "Why regulation fails," Harper's Magazine 251, 16 (September, 1975).

becoming over-regulated? Which are more effective, pre-injury preventive actions or post-injury remedies, and what should "effective" mean? Should some of the matters now in the purview of regulatory agencies be left to the courts? If indeed regulation (or court action) is too clumsy, slow, inflexible, costly, and restraining to the spirit of free enterprise, what are the alternatives?

We will mention three alternatives to government control. The first is voluntary establishment of standards by trade associations and similar groups. This activity, though not familiar to much of the public, is exceedingly important. Most products in the United States are affected by such control, if not in the designing of the products themselves, at least in standardization of the quality of their components. There are many voluntary standards organizations, such as the American Society for Testing and Materials, the American National Standards Institute, Underwriters Laboratories, and the National Fire Protection Association. The scope of this work is such that the American Society for Testing and Materials (ASTM), which calls itself "the world's largest private standards-writing body," has 22,000 members and publishes a 31,000-page *Annual Book of ASTM Standards* describing in technical detail 4,300 individual standards for steel, glass, acoustical materials, fuels, textiles, skid resistant surfaces, surgical implants, and other items that directly affect personal safety.[153]

On a smaller scale, as one example among many, the Crayon, Water Color and Craft Institute, Inc., representing about 80 percent of the industry in such products as children's crayons, chalk, tempera paints, school pastes, finger paints, and block printing inks, develops industry-wide toxicity standards. Products meeting its standards, set by professional toxicologists, are allowed to carry a certifying seal. To give an example of the sort of influence such an organization has, in 1968 it responded to evidence of toxicity of some commonly used phenolic preservatives by requiring its members to eliminate them from their products; over the next four years substitutes were found and the phenolics entirely replaced. The Institute works with the National Bureau of Standards to develop national standards.[154]

We will return to the subjects of standards and certification later. Before moving on, we should point out that voluntary establishment of

---

[153]American Society for Testing and Materials, "ASTM and the voluntary standards system" (1970).

[154]Personal communication, Elizabeth B. Clarkson, executive vice president, The Crayon, Water Color and Craft Institute, Inc.

standards may be conducted in close cooperation with the government, perhaps even under strong advice from the government agency involved. Advisory committees influence the proceedings. Although compliance is voluntary, it may on occasion be made plain that unless the industry improves its products the government will move in and set enforceable standards. This widespread hybrid industry-government strategy deserves intensive evaluation; its effectiveness at actually keeping the public safe, its cost-effectiveness, and its desirability as an alternative or adjunct to tight government control need to be examined critically. Also, since voluntary standards-setting depends upon deliberation by committees of technical people, its implications for professional ethical conduct need to be spelled out.

A second alternative to government regulation—one which directly affects product demand—is private certification by organizations such as Consumers Union and the Good Housekeeping Seal of Approval program. These groups are quite influential. By giving approval to particular products and by issuing warnings of hazards, they influence consumers' buying and manufacturers' output. Some of these organizations are associated with widely-read publications, which serve over the years to heighten the purchasing sensibilities of consumers. In this certifying category we should also mention such industry-associated groups as Underwriters Laboratories, Inc., which certify such wares as electrical items, and the public interest groups that campaign against particular products. Sometimes such organizations take the federal regulatory establishment to task directly, as when in recent years Consumers Union has petitioned the Food and Drug Administration to take action on microwave ovens and on evaporated milk containing traces of lead from soldered can seams.[155]

A third alternative to government regulation is direct consumer action. Recent years have brought a revival of this activity which in earlier times—as people simply patronized, admonished, or boycotted their tradesmen neighbors—had a strong and unbuffered influence on product quality. People are now exploring the use of consumer petition, boycott, legal suit, service on industry and government advisory panels, consumer education, worker retraining, and counter-advertising. The trend is healthy, and avenues of influence are being opened that will prove advantageous to both consumers and industry.

---

[155]Elin Schoen, "*Consumer Reports* knows what's best for us all," *Esquire*, 108 (February 1974).

CRITERIA AND STANDARDS

The boundary between fact and value may be sharpened by distinguishing *criteria* from *standards.* In general, criteria are *descriptive* factors taken into account in setting standards. Standards are *prescriptive* norms established by some authority to govern action. Standards are established in the perspective of criteria. Metaphorically, criteria are appropriately ruled measuring sticks by which hazards are gauged when standards are established.

For example, the Health, Education, and Welfare Department's document, *Air Quality Criteria for Sulfur Oxides,* establishes criteria for the states to take into account in developing their standards governing these common pollutants from combustion of fossil fuels. Stating that "Air quality criteria are an expression of the scientific knowledge of the relationship between various concentrations of pollutants in the air and their adverse effects on man and his environment," the report describes the physical and chemical properties of the sulfur oxides and methods for measuring them; it surveys concentrations of sulfur oxides in the national environment; it reviews the effects of these substances on materials, vegetation, animals, and man (including synergistic effects with particulate matter); and it summarizes the epidemiological record. In other words, the report describes the factors that are judged to be most important. This is principally a scientific document, although some subjective, social value judgments are implicit in it. It does not set any standards.[156]

Standards may be of several types:

Personal exposure standards (example: radiation exposure standards, noise limits)

Ambient composition standards (water quality standards)

Product design standards (seat belt specifications, railroad car coupler standards)

Product composition standards (food composition standards, pewter alloy standards)

Product performance standards (automotive emission standards, mattress flammability limits)

Work practice standards (limitations on air traffic controller work hours, factory temperature standards)

---

[156]U. S. Department of Health, Education, and Welfare, "Air quality criteria for sulfur oxides." National Air Pollution Control Administration Publication No. AP-50 (April, 1970).

Promotional claims standards (drug and cosmetic advertising standards)

Packaging standards (childproof pill-package standards, standards for construction of pressurized gas cylinders).

Although this list is neither exhaustive nor rigorous, it includes most types of standards governing everyday hazards.

This can be said to be the "Age of Numerical Standards." We almost reflexively resort to setting hard-and-fast standards, often under regulation, to resolve our problems. This may not be bad, although in some ways it is too early to know. How does the establishment of standards affect market and product development flexibility? Are standards mechanisms cost-effective? Which are more efficient and effective in the long run, voluntary industry standards or government standards? What incentives are there for voluntary action?

Some standards are remarkably detailed and precise. The Consumer Product Safety Commission, described by one observer as engaging in "regulation by the numbers," has, for example, ruled that in order to prevent babies from strangling in cribs, "the distance between components (such as slats, spindles, crib rods, and corner posts) shall not be greater than 2⅜ inches at any point." That spacing was derived from measurements of many babies, and supposedly will protect more than 95 percent of all American infants.[157] Mattresses must now pass flammability tests with lighted "cigarettes without filter tips made from natural tobacco, 85 ± 2 mm long with a tobacco packing density of 0.270 ± 0.020 g/cm^3 and a total weight of 1.1 ± 0.1 g" in a test room warmer than 65° F., with relative humidity less than 55 percent. A specified number of the char tests must be made on sample mattresses, which pass if they char around each cigarette no more than 2 inches.[158] The Commission has proposed detailed design and performance specifications for bicycles, including such provisions as "the tensile strength of the drive chain shall be no less than 1800 lb ... The manufacturer's recommended inflation pressure shall be molded into or onto the sidewall of the tire with lettering no less than

[157]U.S. Consumer Product Safety Commission, "Requirements for baby cribs," *21 U. S. Code of Federal Regulations,* 191e; the crib standard is discussed in Steven Kelman, "Regulation by the numbers—a report on the Consumer Product Safety Commission," *The Public Interest 36,* 83-102 (1974).

[158]U. S. Consumer Product Safety Commission, "Mattresses. Notice of amendments to flammability standards," *38 Federal Register,* 15095-15101 (June 8, 1973).

[159]U. S. Consumer Product Safety Commission, "Establishment of safety standards and proposed labelling requirements for bicycles," *39 Federal Register,* 26100-26112 (July 16, 1974).

3.2 mm (⅛ in.) in height . . . Each pedal shall have reflectors located on the front and rear surfaces of the pedal . . ."[159]

The key question is whether such regulation will be effective *in preventing injuries*. With bicycles, is the physical design of the product really the problem? Or is it rider carelessness, poorly maintained street surfaces, poor provision of cycle lanes, or lack of general public acceptance of bicycles? What are the most cost-effective ways of reducing injury to bicycle riders?[160]

A few years from now we shall have to submit "regulation by the numbers" to evaluation by the numbers (of risks reduced, costs paid, and so on) in order to determine how efficient, how effective, how equitable, and how costly these protective measures have been.

Developing criteria independently of standards is becoming a widespread practice, as in the sulfur oxides case described above, and in the Environmental Protection Agency's management of noise control. In occupational safety, criteria and standards are kept separate by assigning their development to two different agencies: the National Institute of Occupational Safety and Health (NIOSH, of the Department of Health, Education and Welfare) develops criteria, whereas the Occupational Safety and Health Administration (OSHA, of the Labor Department) sets standards guided by the criteria proposed by NIOSH.[161]

Rarely is a level of risk *first* decided upon as acceptable *before* exposure is limited in order to keep the hazard down to the level agreed upon. For chemical carcinogens, attempts have been made to set maximum "acceptable risk doses" which can be expected to assure "virtual safety" at some preselected hazard level (say, one tumor per hundred million people exposed).[162] The task is difficult but, in theory, appealing. The Food and Drug Administration has used this approach in setting tolerances for residues of the carcinogenic cattle growth hormone diethylstilbestrol

[159]U. S. Consumer Product Safety Commission, "Establishment of safety standards and proposed labelling requirements for bicycles," *39 Federal Register*, 26100-26112 (July 16, 1974).

[160]For general commentary on the Consumer Product Safety Commission's work, see Paul H. Weaver, "The hazards of trying to make consumer products safer," *Fortune 42*, #1, 133-140 (July, 1975).

[161]U. S. Environmental Protection Agency, *Public Health and Welfare Criteria for Noise*, EPA 550/9-73-002 (July 27, 1973); U. S. National Institute of Occupational Safety and Health, *Criteria for a Recommended Standard . . . Occupational Exposure to Inorganic Lead* (1972).

[162]Nathan Mantel and W. Raye Bryan, " 'Safety' testing of carcinogenic agents," *Journal of the National Cancer Institute 27*, 455-470 (1961); Ad Hoc Committee on the Evaluation of Low Levels of Environmental Chemical Carcinogens, "Evaluation of environmental carcinogens—Report to the Surgeon General, USPHS," in the *Congressional Record*, E952-958 (February 9, 1972).

(DES), and the Environmental Protection Agency has used it in setting chemical plant effluent standards for benzidine, another carcinogen.[163] As reported in *Science,*

> For benzidine, officials in the agency's Office of Toxic Substances began by selecting a risk that seemed acceptable—a chance of one in a million that people drinking water contaminated with benzidine would develop cancer—and then calculated a "dose" or exposure limit that would pose a risk of cancer no greater than this. The Environmental Protection Agency based its calculations on small-scale rat experiments done in the late 1950s that showed benzidine to be a carcinogen in mammals. To account for the differences between rats and men, and for a number of other imponderables, the Environmental Protection Agency threw in a safety factor of 100 and ended up with a standard that—if formally adopted—would allow dye manufacturers to dispose of no more than a pound of benzidine a day in a moderately large river flowing at 10,000 cubic feet per second.[164]

The degree to which safety judgments are relative is obvious if one compares criteria and standards from several nations. Radiation exposure standards differ widely from country to country, as do pharmaceutical and environmental standards.[165]

In a significant recent development, the courts have ruled that the setting of federal occupational exposure standards can take into account the economic feasibility of the standards. Ruling on an aspect of the Occupational Safety and Health Administration's asbestos dust standard, the court noted that "practical considerations can temper protective requirements. Congress does not appear to have intended to protect employees by putting their employers out of business ... It would comport with common usage to say that a standard that is prohibitively expensive is not 'feasible' ... We conclude that the factors entering into the Secretary of Labor's conclusion could properly include problems of economic feasibility." This principle is likely to be carried over into other areas.[166]

---

[163]U. S. Food and Drug Administration, Compounds used in food-producing animals, *38 Federal Register,* 19226-19230 (July 19, 1973); U. S. Environmental Protection Agency, "Proposed toxic pollutant effluent standards," *38 Federal Register,* 35388-35395 (December 27, 1973), and *39 Federal Register,* 3756-3797 (January 29, 1974).

[164]Robert Gillette, "Cancer and the environment II: groping for new remedies," *Science 186,* 242-245 (1974).

[165]World Health Organization, *Health Hazards of the Human Environment,* 134 (WHO, Geneva, 1972).

[166]Industrial Union Department, AFL-CIO v. James D. Hodgson, Secretary, Department of Labor, U. S. Court of Appeals, District of Columbia Circuit (April 15, 1974) in *Federal Reporter* 499 F2d 467 (1974).

MAKING PRODUCTS SAFE

One has only to scan such statistics as those cited by the final report of the National Commission on Product Safety to be struck by the magnitude of product-related injuries:

Every year, about 150,000 victims of broken windows, doors, or glass walls discover that what they can't see can hurt them. About 100,000 walked through glass doors last year [1968], probably believing the space to be open ... Among the 85 million TV sets in the United States in 1969, including about 20 million color sets, about 10,000 caught fire ... Lacking effective guards against whirling gears, chains, teeth, blades, or flying fragments and without effective insulation against high voltage, some power tools are menacing. They are responsible for injuring more than 125,000 do-it-yourselfers every year ... The U. S. Public Health Service estimates that toys injure 70,000 children every year ...[167]

Similarly, "there are annually [as of 1972] 3,000 to 5,000 deaths and 150,000 to 250,000 injuries from burns associated with flammable fabrics."[168] From explosions of pressurized beer, champagne, and soft drink bottles, "last year alone some 111,000 emergency room cases were associated with glass containers."[169] Many of the 55,000 annual motor vehicle deaths and 2,000,000 disabling injuries from automobiles are caused by mechanical failures in the vehicles themselves. The casualty list could go on and on.

No doubt many of these accidents were due to error on the part of the users. But in general we expect manufacturers to reduce the problem by making their products as safe as is reasonable. Among other considerations, that reasonableness implies anticipating misuse and the vulnerabilities of especially sensitive persons. A manufacturer of children's products—blocks, rattles, sweaters, anything—who does not anticipate that sooner or later they will be chewed on, thrown at playmates, rubbed against the face, and otherwise treated the way infants just naturally treat

---

[167]National Commission on Product Safety, *Final Report*, 12-31 (1970).

[168]U. S. Department of Health, Education, and Welfare, *Flammable Fabrics*, vi, (1972).

[169]Hearings on glass containers by the Consumer Product Safety Commission in April 1974, reported in "The exploding bottle case," *Washington Post* (April 18, 1974).

things, is morally, if not legally, negligent. In the same way, a manufacturer of an antihistamine that can make some people drowsy would be negligent not to print a warning of that possibility on the package.

The concepts of negligence and reasonableness pervade the law with respect to consumer product safety. Legally, negligence is usually defined as "conduct which involves an unreasonably great risk of damage." In general, the common law holds people to standards of what reasonably prudent persons would do in the circumstances. Under the law, reasonableness is determined by such factors as the probability of harm, the seriousness of the risk, the social value of the interests involved, and the availability of alternatives.[170] Considering the diversity of views people might hold in judging a hazard by these criteria, it is no wonder that judges deciding claims of liability for product-associated injuries often prefer to relegate the question of reasonableness to a jury![171]

Safeguarding actions are possible at every stage in the formative life of products, beginning with design and moving through certification or licensing, to manufacturing quality control, packaging and labelling, and on through advertising and marketing. And then products can be followed onto the market to monitor safety in use.

Designing

Products receive their initial shaping at the hand of designers and development engineers. Corners are given their sharpness on the drawing board. Materials are specified in the development laboratory. During the development of a product, technical and marketing specialists advise on what will sell: power saws with blade guards, or without; insulation on an electrical component, or no insulation; a safety lock, or a warning label, or a protective cover, or a flame-retardant finish, or non-allergenic ingredients.

In the design process, questions are asked about what might possibly happen during use of the product. An agricultural engineer has listed some typical questions pertaining to the design of farm equipment: "How much weight should an operator be expected to lift when hitching an implement to a tractor? What are acceptable sound levels for farm equipment? How

---

[170]Michael J. Wollan, "The process of setting safety standards in the courts, Congress, and administrative agencies," staff discussion paper no. 204, George Washington University Program of Policy Studies in Science and Technology, National Technical Information Service PB 182 876 (1968).

[171]See also p. 116ff.

do you design and orient chemical applicating equipment so an operator isn't unduly exposed to chemicals or vapors when loading or adjusting the machine? How much time does an operator need for taking corrective action when he senses his tractor is about to tip over?"[172]

"Human factors engineering," the field which specifically attempts to tailor products to the physical and mental capabilities of their users, would answer the above questions about farm equipment design by taking into account measurements of operator strengths and body dimensions, noise exposure-effect relations, and reaction times. Although tractor design has evolved over the years to incorporate many important safety features, still about a thousand deaths and many more injuries are inflicted annually in agricultural tractor accidents. The Department of Transportation recently listed the most important safeguarding features available for tractors: overturn-protective frames similar to automobile "roll bars"; hydraulic self-equalizing brakes to compensate, in road use, for unequal wear on the rear wheel brakes, which operate independently to assist in making tight turns and which are worn unequally in repetitive end-of-row turns in one direction; shielding of the power-takeoff shaft to accessories; safer arrangements for making wheel-spacing adjustments; use of less flammable diesel fuel instead of gasoline; removal of the fuel tank from the vicinity of the engine, which may act as an ignition source; and wide-front-axle configurations instead of the older, less stable, tricycle designs.[173] Measurements of body dimensions have led to improved seat design; acoustic analyses have led to muffling and deflection of noise; and observations of operator habits and reactions have led to better placement and design of controls.

Similarly in a different area, the National Bureau of Standards has recently completed studies of children's body measurements and strengths for the purpose of guiding the design of children's toys and other products.[174] Research is needed on women's strength and physiological response to stress, for as more women move into what have been strictly men's occupations they will encounter what are for them new hazards. One suspects that much of the regulation and design for women's

---

[172]Page L. Bellinger, "Man-machine compatibility," *Agricultural Engineering 50*, 17-19 (January 1969).

[173]U. S. Secretary of Transportation, *Agricultural Tractor Safety on Public Roads and Farms*, a report to the Congress (January 1971).

[174]U. S. National Bureau of Standards: "A study of the strength capabilities of children, aged 2-6," NBS IR 73-156 (August 1973), and "A study of young children's pull-apart strength," NBS IR 73-424 (April 1974).

occupational safety has been based on guess, hearsay, and old-foremen's-tales. The techniques of investigation are readily available; many of them have been developed thoroughly by the military and by the National Aeronautics and Space Administration.

Product designing has become a very technical profession, with much design work being done by teams. But in essence it is still a matter of common sense—asking over and over, "What can go wrong? What can possibly, by any accident, go wrong?" And then, "What can be done to prevent that?"

One example of neglectful design was pointed out by a group of architects who recently reviewed the literature on the design of stairs. They found that "it turns out to consist largely of empirical rules of thumb. No one seems to have examined closely the sense of comfort or strain, safety or danger that the user experiences in climbing or descending a particular kind of stairway." The investigators, whose attention was attracted in part by the large number of nighttime falls on the four broad, shallow, unmarked steps in front of the Metropolitan Opera House in New York, have now studied stairs extensively and have made recommendations for improving their design.[175]

As an example of a product whose design has been considerably improved through the years, we might mention automobile safety glazing. The plate glass that had so glamorously replaced flapping curtains, plain window glass, and isinglass soon turned out to be responsible for 45 percent of all the injuries incurred in automobile accidents. Its sharp fragments scattered and cut like shrapnel. Laminated safety glass (which tradition says was discovered when someone dropped a test tube containing the plastic, cellulose nitrate, and the tube broke but did not fly apart) was developed for windshields about 1927; an interlayer of plastic bonded between two glass sheets keeps the glass from shattering badly. Further improvements in tempering (heat treating) and laminating, to provide an even more tolerable mode of breakage and more resistance to penetration by a person's head, have since become standard.[176]

Designing large, complex structures obviously calls for extraordinarily sophisticated approaches. But even on thoroughly analyzed projects, such

---

[175]James Marston Fitch, John Templer, and Paul Corcoran, "The dimensions of stairs," *Scientific American* 231, 82-91 (October, 1974).

[176]"Operation windshield," *Standardization 21*, 144-151 (1950); "New safety glazing code = greater protection for vehicle users," *The Magazine of Standards 37*, 328-330 (1966).

as the Bay Area Rapid Transit system, hazards can still be overlooked.[177] Our loss of three astronauts on the ground at Cape Kennedy demonstrated that even the best no-cost-spared systems-analytic approaches in the world cannot anticipate every possibility.

Developmental Testing

When prototypes become available from the development laboratory they are usually subjected to some kind of simulated-use testing or "proving out." Their safety, among other qualities, is evaluated. Vulnerable points of the design are reviewed. For products such as chemical preparations, tests are performed on animals. For pharmaceuticals, medical devices, and other products with deep physiological implications, tests are eventually done on humans if preliminary animal tests are encouraging. Automobiles are driven on test tracks. Electrical equipment is overloaded and subjected to heat, cold, and vibration.

Certifying and Licensing

At a fairly advanced stage in development, certification may be sought; for instance, approval from Underwriters Laboratories might be requested for an electrical switchbox. Government licensing may be required. A new drug must be approved by the Food and Drug Administration prior to marketing, so the manufacturer pursues an application in which he provides evidence to Food and Drug Administration examiners that his product is both safe and efficacious under the conditions for which its use is prescribed. The burden of proof is on the manufacturer. The process is intensive in scientific detail, legally complex, slow, and very expensive. The manufacturer adjusts his product development pace to the Food and Drug Administration's recommendations about the required animal and human testing. The process is reiterative: testing, review, more testing. Eventually, if the product is judged to be of acceptable efficacy and risk by both the manufacturer and the Food and Drug Administration, and if it promises to make a great enough profit for the manufacturer over a long enough term, it goes on the market.

---

[177]Charles G. Burck, "What we can learn from BART's misadventures," *Fortune 42,* no. 1, 104ff. (July, 1975).

Controlling Quality

Supervising the fidelity of individual items to design specifications as they come off the assembly line is the next influence on products' quality. Failure of items to conform to specifications—because of tool error, error of assembly, defective starting materials, contamination, or careless finishing—obviously undoes all the cautious work of development. The quality control task, easily overlooked as unglamorous, is both difficult and critical. It takes just one inadequately sterilized can of soup retaining viable *botulinus* spores to cause serious illness, one batch of contaminated eye makeup ingredients to cause many eye infections, one faulty brake part to cause an accident. Vigilance, a numbing vigilance, is called for to give adequate inspection to the hypnotizingly similar items streaming down a production line. Automated methods can help, as can the principles of sampling and performance testing. Dramatic development of both mechanical and statistical testing techniques by the aerospace and other high-technology industries, prodded by exhortations from the "consumer movement," have heightened emphasis on quality control, and quality control engineering has become a highly respected profession.[178]

Packaging and Labelling

As products are readied for sale another possibility for making safe comes in packaging and in providing instructions and special warnings. In recent years we have seen striking changes in packaging, not all of them desirable. The chemical industry has benefitted greatly in its own operations from using shatterproof plastic and rubber containers, in place of glass ones, for industrial chemicals; it now provides similar, smaller containers for some of its more hazardous household products.

The controversy that can arise over packaging is neatly exemplified by the seemingly simple issue of "childproof" containers. In 1970 Congress passed the Poison Prevention Packaging Act (Public Law 91-601) which requires that special safety packaging be provided for certain household poisons. (Note that a few manufacturers had already voluntarily taken steps in this direction). Responsibility for administration of the act was assigned to the Consumer Product Safety Commission, which has now set requirements for safety caps on a number of household products such as aspirin, turpentine, amphetamines, barbiturates, and lye.

---

[178]Joseph M. Juran and F. M. Gryna, *Quality Planning and Analysis: From Product Development through Usage* (McGraw-Hill, New York, 1970).

A detailed protocol for testing has been established: for each package design, the packages are to be given for five minutes to 200 children (in pairs) between the ages of 42 and 51 months, with instructions to try to open the package. After the five-minute period, the demonstrator opens the package once and tells the children that they may use their teeth. The children are then given another five minutes to work. If no more than 15 percent of the children open the package before the demonstration and no more than 20 percent do after it, the package passes this part of the test.[179] Informal estimates are that the safety closures cost a penny or so more than conventional lids. The Congress obviously thought the plan reasonable, and the agency has proceeded carefully in enforcing it, but the plan has many vocal opponents. They complain that the lids are too difficult even for adults to manage, that the cost increase is intolerable, that children quickly learn to open them anyway, and that the whole matter is not the government's business in the first place. In a similar effort, Great Britain is now adopting individual-wrapping nonreclosable-package plans calling for plastic blister or paper strip packages for aspirin and other pills. In a few years it will be essential to determine whether there has been a significant decrease in poisoning because of the new regulations, which in the meantime will probably be extended to other household chemicals.

Products are often provided with detailed directions for use and with warning labels. Pesticides for farm and home use; cosmetics and toiletries such as dandruff-preventive shampoos and lotions containing steroids; proprietary drugs; power tools and household appliances such as lathes and meat grinders; toys such as darts and chemistry sets—all of these may carry warnings against misuse, instructions for proper use, injunctions against letting children use them, or admonitions to discontinue use if adverse reactions occur. Such directions are helpful, and manufacturers would be negligent not to provide them. But labels alone cannot prevent improper use. One need only think of the Surgeon General's warning cited on every pack of cigarettes. As surveys have shown, and as is confirmed by everyday experience, people frequently—perhaps usually—ignore warning labels.[180]

Other kinds of labelling contribute to safety. Recent hearings on the safety of cosmetics brought forth recommendations that labels on cosmetics,

---

[179]*21 U. S. Code of Federal Regulations*, 295.

[180]A. C. Miller, Arnold Mallis, and W. C. Easterlin, "Do people read labels on household insecticides?" *Soap and Chemical Specialties 34*, no. 7, 61-63 (1958).

perfumes, and toiletries carry lists of ingredients, employ such designations as "hypoallergenic" with as much uniformity and precision as possible, and carry discontinuation dates for perishable ingredients. These precautions are meant to prevent allergic reactions and eye infections. The debate is an intense one, involving several billion dollars' worth of products.[181]

Sometimes it is possible, at very low cost, to incorporate into a product an effective warning feature which can hardly be overlooked. We think of such devices as the trace of brilliant fluorescein dye sometimes added to poisonous wood alcohol to deter people from drinking it, the warning dyes incorporated into fungicidal seed coatings, and the trace of repulsive-smelling sulfur compound added to otherwise almost odorless natural gas supplies to warn of gas leaks.

Advertising

As we know from the turn-of-the-century patent medicine manufacturer's unrestrained claims that frequent use of their laxatives was the key to "regularity," advertisements definitely can induce people to take higher risks.

What is not so clear is how successful advertising is at fostering *safe* practices. A panel of the National Advertising Review Board recently recommended that in advertisements "users should not be shown on the top step of a ladder," and that "children or pets should not be nearby when power equipment is in use." The panel concluded that "advertising can do more than it is now doing to safeguard the users of advertised products without impairing its ability to merchandise those products effectively."[182]

Following onto the Market

Products can be followed onto the market to judge their safety as well as other characteristics. Epidemiological studies, monitoring and surveillance, and accident case investigations can reveal previously unsuspected design faults, performance failure, misuse, and unsuspected adverse effects.

Some manufacturers are quite responsible in following their products onto the market and improving them in the light of what is learned. Others do little or nothing. The "consumer movement," tightening of government

---

[181]U. S. Senate Committee on Labor and Public Welfare, Subcommittee on Health, *Hearings on the Cosmetic Safety Act of 1974* (February 20 and 21, 1974).

[182]Consultative panel of the National Advertising Review Board, "Product advertising and consumer safety," (June, 1974).

regulations, sterner court attitudes about liability, and the emergence of product safety as a selling point have all encouraged manufacturers to pay more attention to the safety of products in use.

There is no "right" balance between screening products before they are marketed, and following them after they are sold. Some products are screened, or filtered, with exceeding care before they get to the general public. In the United States pharmaceuticals have to undergo years of testing on animals and then on people, under close supervision, before they are approved by the Food and Drug Administration and released for general sale by manufacturers. In contrast, some European governments require less premarket testing, and more new drugs are put on the market; but concomitantly, those nations often require rigorous monitoring in order to detect adverse side effects. The question of strategies for managing the introduction of new drugs has always been controversial.

Provocative data were provided recently in a comparative study by University of Rochester pharmacologist William M. Wardell. Examining the period from 1962 to 1971, he found that "nearly four times as many new drugs became exclusively available in Great Britain as in the United States."[183] Further,

> On the evidence currently available, Britain probably did not lose appreciably from the introduction of ineffective drugs, nor from the fact that a greater number of new drugs were made available. The main deleterious effect was that Britain suffered more toxicity due to new drugs than did the United States, as could have been anticipated from the fact that more new drugs were marketed there. However, considering the size of the total burden of drug toxicity, the portion due to new drugs was extremely small, and would in any case be at least partially offset by the adverse effects of older alternative drugs had the latter been used instead. Conversely, Britain experiences clearly discernible gains by introducing useful new drugs, either sooner than the United States or exclusively. On balance, Britain appears to have gained in comparison from its more permissive policy toward the marketing of new drugs coupled with a more rigorous program of postmarketing surveillance.[184]

Wardell's studies are being reviewed currently; it will be interesting to see how the argument shapes up. The desirability of intensifying postmarketing

---

[183]William M. Wardell, "Introduction of new therapeutic drugs in the United States and Great Britain: an international comparison," Clinical Pharmacology and Therapeutics 14, 773-790 (1973).

[184]William M. Wardell, "Therapeutic implication of the drug lag," Clinical Pharmacology and Therapeutics 15, 73-96 (1974).

surveillance, perhaps even at the expense of relaxing premarketing testing a bit, is being championed in several quarters.[185]

MAKING THE GENERAL ENVIRONMENT SAFE

Because we have discussed environmental hazards such as noise, lead, radiation, and DDT extensively elsewhere in this report, because good analyses of environmental hazards are available, and because many of the problems resemble the product safety problems just discussed, we will simply summarize here a few special features of environmental safety.[186]

Environmental hazards are diffuse and difficult to analyze. Moved around as they are by the currents of air and water, even their physical presence is hard to appraise. Many are invisible and odorless. Many of the hazards, such as noise, work their effects so slowly that the victims are usually in their later years and are restrained by long habit from moving away or making an active protest, and the people too young to have suffered from cumulative effect have little personal motivation to do anything about the threat. As we have pointed out, environmental problems are often attacked by means of government regulation.

A special environmental problem is occupational safety, to which we now turn.

MAKING THE WORKPLACE SAFE

The statistics are appalling:

Three and a half million American workers exposed to asbestos face a dual threat: not only are they subject to the lung-scarring pneumoconiosis of their trade, *asbestosis*, but are endangered by *lung cancer* associated with inhalation

---

[185]An evaluation which finds that enforcement of the 1962 drug efficacy legislation "seems to have generated sizeable net benefits for consumers" appears in James Marshall Jondrow, *A Measure of the Monetary Benefits and Costs to Consumers of the Regulation of Prescription Drug Effectiveness*, Ph.D. dissertation, University of Wisconsin, 1972, available as facsimile 72-27,332 from University Microfilms, Inc., Ann Arbor, Michigan; see also Robert B. Helms, editor, *Drug Development and Marketing*, the report of a conference held in July, 1974, by the American Enterprise Institute for Public Policy Research, 1150 Seventeenth Street, Washington, D. C. 20036.

[186]Three good general texts are Barbara Ward and René Dubos, *Only One Earth* (W. W. Norton and Co., New York, 1972); George L. Waldbott, *Health Effects of Environmental Pollutants* (C. V. Mosby Co., St. Louis, 1973); and World Health Organization, *Health Hazards of the Human Environment* (WHO, Geneva, 1972).

of asbestos fibers. Recent studies of insulation workers in two states showed 1 in 5 deaths were from lung cancer, 7 times the expected rate; half of those with 20 years or more in the trade had X-ray evidence of *asbestosis*; 1 in 10 deaths were caused by *mesothelioma*, a rare malignancy of the lung or pleura which strikes only 1 in 10,000 in the general working population.

Of 6,000 men who have been uranium miners, an estimated 600 to 1,100 will die during the next 20 years as a result of *radiation exposure*, principally from lung cancer.

Fifty percent of the machines in industry generate *noise* levels potentially harmful to hearing.

Hundreds of thousands of workers each year suffer skin diseases from contact with materials used in their work. The *dermatoses* are the most common of all occupational illnesses.

Even the old, well-known industrial poisons, such as mercury, arsenic, and lead, still cause trouble. In New Mexico recently, workers dismantling a missile site were hospitalized from *lead intoxication* after using acetylene torches to cut structural steel coated with a red lead paint.[187]

Every year among our 75,000,000 employed civilians there are at least 336,000 cases of occupationally related disease. In addition to disease, accidents on the job annually cause more than 14,200 deaths and 2,500,000 disabling injuries.[188]

Extreme heat and cold; noisy, vibrating machinery; rock dust, textile fiber dust, flour dust; chemical fumes; mercury, lead, beryllium, arsenic; corrosives, poisons, skin irritants, radiation—these all assail workers, in addition to the more obvious hazards of mechanical injury, burns, and electrocution.

Much can be done to make workplaces safe. Ventilating, restraining, shielding, and warning equipment can be installed. Protective clothing, hair nets, respirators, ear protectors, and goggles can be provided, as can emergency equipment such as gas masks, first aid supplies, and firefighting tools. Training workers to work carefully and to anticipate hazards is particularly important; ignorance, absentmindedness, negligence, and foolhardiness are the precipitating factors in a large proportion of industrial accidents. The rest result from mechanical faults such as defective parts, damaged electric cables, and worn-out hoisting ropes, and unguarded machines.[189]

---

[187]U. S. Department of Health, Education, and Welfare, "Occupational disease . . . The silent enemy".

[188]National Safety Council, *Accident Facts* (1974).

[189]International Labour Office, *Accident Prevention: A Worker's Education Manual* (ILO, Geneva, 1972).

Industry associations campaign for improvement of worker protection, as do labor unions. Recently, public interest groups have played catalytic roles. Broad regulatory power has been given to the Labor Department's Occupational Safety and Health Administration (OSHA) by the Occupational Safety and Health Act of 1970 (Public Law 91-596).[190] It is too early yet to judge what impact OSHA will have. The Administration has already been challenged by several issues, including a difficult one regarding conditions for exposure to certain carcinogenic chemicals in industry. OSHA is currently confronting major questions about asbestos, arsenic, and vinyl chloride, each of which may possibly affect more than a million workers each; its effectiveness in dealing with these initial problems will help determine the agency's future importance. Once again, society is relying on regulation to solve the problems; again, the effectiveness of that strategy begs to be evaluated.[191]

The need for research on occupational safety has been publicized repeatedly. As the firm of Arthur D. Little, Inc. has summarized the reseach scene,[192]

> Research in traffic and vehicular safety, fire and explosion safety hazards and mine safety (mostly fire and explosion) far outweigh the effort devoted to other occupational safety research. During the 1940s and 50s much work on fatigue, working stress, and human factors design of machines was conducted—much of this was done by the Department of Defense and the Atomic Energy Commission. Continuation of this effort by the National Aeronautics and Space Administration has been significant, but the total effort has decreased in the last ten years. Research in ergonomics (the matching of machines to men), motivation and psychological aspects of safety continues at a low level, primarily at universities. Several of the large state universities have on-going projects in farm safety, and several universities and federal agencies are conducting research on accident investigation techniques. Formal research in safety equipment, criteria and standards development, physical safety and accident causative factors seems to be limited.[193]

---

[190]*The President's Report on Occupational Safety and Health*, 1972.

[191]U. S. Controller General, "Slow progress likely in development of standards for toxic substances and harmful physical agents found in workplaces," a report to the U. S. Senate Committee on Labor and Public Welfare (September 28, 1973).

[192]Arthur D. Little, Inc., "The present status and requirements for occupational safety research," prepared for the National Institute for Occupational Safety and Health, HEW, on contract no. HSM 099-71-30 (1972).

[193]General discussion appears in D. Hunter, *The Diseases of Occupations* (English Universities Press, London, 1955); May R. Mayers, *Occupational Health: Hazards of the Work Environment* (Williams and

MAKING SAFE THROUGH EDUCATION

Although the estimates vary widely, it is generally agreed that a majority of accidents, and a large number of illnesses, are in some sense the direct result of ignorance or carelessness on the part of those exposed. We have all known people who have done it, or we have done it ourselves: fallen off a bicycle, driven sleepily off the road, caught a finger or hair in a whirling tool or home appliance, fallen down stairs, gotten hurt while taking a short-cut or circumventing a safeguard, or carelessly started a fire.

In some hazard areas we do train people to avoid danger. School programs train automobile drivers and, in some rural areas, tractor and farm equipment operators. Occupational training programs usually include some discussion of safe practices in the use of tools and some training for response to emergencies. Military and industrial on-site training stresses safety.

In the past few years, school, public interest, government, and corporation consumer education programs have been instituted to help consumers take care of themselves. Some of these programs aim to influence the public's purchasing decisions; some catalyze influence on government and industrial decisions; some train for safe use of products.[194]

Most current regulatory programs concentrate on product quality and other determinants of safety rather than on user behavior. However, there are exceptions: the Poison Control Centers issue public warnings of household poisoning dangers, and the Consumer Product Safety Commission publicizes the hazardous features of toys. In many areas we need to ask whether expending more effort on education might be an effective way of making safe. And existing educational programs, which often seem ineffective, need to be evaluated.

MONITORING AND SURVEILLANCE

For present purposes we will adopt the World Health Organization's definitions.[195]

Wilkins, Baltimore, 1969); *The President's Report on Occupational Safety and Health*, 1972; Franklin Wallick; *The American Worker: An Endangered Species* (Ballantine, New York, 1972); Jeanne M. Stellman and Susan Daum, *Work is Dangerous to your Health* (Pantheon, New York, 1973); Paul Brodeur, *Expendable Americans* (Viking, New York, 1974); Rachel Scott, *Muscle and Blood* (Dutton, New York, 1974); Nicholas A. Ashford, "Crisis in the workplace: Occupational disease and injury," a report to the Ford Foundation (MIT Press, Cambridge, 1975).

[194]A recent example of a public interest "how-to" effort is Priscilla W. Laws, *Medical and dental X-rays: A consumer's guide to avoiding unnecessary radiation exposure* (Public Citizen/Health Research Group, November, 1974).

[195]World Health Organization, *Health Hazards of the Human Environment*, 269 (WHO, Geneva, 1972).

Monitoring is the making of routine observations on health and environmental parameters, and the recording and transmission of these data.

Health surveillance is the collation and interpretation of data collected from monitoring programmes and from any other available sources, with a view to the detection of changes in health status of populations.

As we learn how to view the world as a network of larger and larger systems, all of which influence each other, and as we develop ways to analyze those systems, monitoring and surveillance become more important. Our major successes so far have probably been in monitoring air and water quality and in maintaining surveillance of the principal causes of death. In the last few years many proposals and programs have been instituted to keep tabs on the quality of the environment.

Air quality and *water quality* are monitored continually by the network of stations of the Environmental Protection Agency.

The National Cancer Institute is updating our knowledge of *cancer incidence* in its "Third National Cancer Survey," gathering data on the incidence of various forms of cancer from hospitals, clinics, laboratories, vital statistics officers, and selected physicians in seven metropolitan areas, in two states, and in Puerto Rico.[196] Writing about the National Cancer Institute study, Philip Abelson, the editor of *Science*, argued for its importance, urging that "surveillance should be continuous, not spasmodic, and it should exploit the power of an electronic computer network. If epidemiologists are to make optimum progress in identifying environmental hazards, they need to be alerted when symptoms first appear and not some years later, after the victims have died."[197]

The need for *clinical drug surveillance* was presented by a report on the general anesthetic, halothane:

In the history of medicine, it is doubtful whether any drug was ever more extensively studied both before and after its introduction than halothane. Yet, after halothane had been given to patients 10 million times, it was impossible to give firm, reliable answers to many basic questions about its effects. Two such questions were: 'How does the death rate after operations under halothane anesthesia compare with death rates when other anesthetics are used?' 'Does halothane induce significantly more [liver function impairment] than other widely used anesthetics?' The National Halothane Study attempted to answer

---

[196]National Cancer Institute, *Cancer Facts 1973*; National Cancer Institute, "Third National Cancer Survey, Advanced Three Year Report, 1969-1971 Incidence," DHEW No. NIH 75-637 (1975).

[197]Philip H. Abelson, "Prevention of cancer," *Science 182*, 973 (1973).

these questions by using existing records. Although 856,500 operations were brought under scrutiny the answers given are predictably and regrettably short of those desired . . . The limitations of knowledge on halothane are certainly not peculiar to it. Limitations at least equally compelling apply to nearly any drug introduced in the past.

The report then recommended "the establishment of a cooperating group of institutions to serve as a panel-laboratory for the acquisition of trustworthy information on new drugs (not merely anesthetics) as they come into use."[198]

A large-scale drug surveillance program is now being conducted by a group of hospitals around the country (the Boston Collaborative Drug Surveillance Program). "Specially-trained monitors stationed on medical wards record information on consecutively admitted patients. Data are collected on patient characteristics, diagnoses, therapeutic effects of all drugs, dosage, duration of therapy and adverse reactions."[199] This approach has already proved useful in investigating drugs in clinical use, revealing adverse effects, interactions of various drugs, and other factors that affect the efficacy and toxicity of medicines.

Automotive, home, industrial, and other accidents are monitored by a number of organizations such as the National Safety Council, and by many government agencies.

Accidents involving consumer products are under surveillance by the Consumer Product Safety Commission, established in 1970.[200] Recognizing that little large-scale assessment of the safety of consumer products has been done, the commission has established a National Electronic Injury Surveillance System (NEISS) to monitor admissions to the emergency rooms of 119 large hospitals and compile statistics on accidents involving consumer products. In its first year the system analyzed almost half a million product related injuries. The analyses correlate the kind of product involved with the nature and severity of injury and with the age and sex of the injured persons. Reports have been published on babies' high chairs, matches, swimming pools, flammable fabrics, and many other products. Periodic tabulations of findings are made available.

---

[198]National Academy of Sciences/National Research Council, Subcommittee on the National Halothane Study, *The National Halothane Study*, 418 (National Institutes of Health, 1969).

[199]Russell R. Miller, "Drug surveillance utilizing epidemiologic methods," *American Journal of Hospital Pharmacy 30*, 584-592 (1973); see also J. S. Campbell and E. Napke, "Drug reaction control," *Modern Medicine of Canada 29*, no. 6 (1974).

[200]Consumer Product Safety Act, Public Law 92-573; Philip H. Abelson, "Consumer Product Safety," *Science 179*, 17 (1973).

This is not an appropriate forum in which to discuss the desirability or success of such a controversial, potentially powerful agency. But we would point to this injury analysis as being novel in scale and a test for the notion that such computerized assessments can identify serious hazards in such a way as to indicate protective and remedial priorities.[201]

A *national fire data system* has recently been proposed for the United States, to analyze causes, frequency of occurrence, and consequences of fires. It would gather data continuously from fire-fighting services, hospitals, the insurance industry, and a number of other sources in an attempt to help set priorities for preventing and controlling fires.[202]

Monitoring the human population for *genetic mutation* has so far not been conducted on a large scale. But it has been strongly advocated: "Laboratory screening systems can certainly reduce the chance of serious human exposure (to chemical mutagens). But now that man has created for himself an unnatural and rapidly changing environment, he ought to have wisdom to institute a continuing scan on his own mutation rate. Otherwise, some chemical or combination of chemicals or perhaps a virus that no one knew or thought to test or some mechanism not detectable in laboratory systems may inflict serious damage before it is detected and before its genetic nature is realized."[203]

Technically speaking, some of the above programs are surveys rather than surveillance, in that "surveillance" implies a continuous activity; however, any of them could be converted to ongoing programs. Many other hazards are, or could be, subject to large-scale monitoring.

A quiet word of skepticism: in this data-collecting age, unless monitoring and surveillance programs are exceptionally well planned so as to facilitate the setting of policy (assigning priorities, allocating funds, making rules, and so on), they will be of little use, wasteful, or perhaps even harmful. Decisionmakers are constantly swamped by data. We can't monitor everything. Costs are very high, personal privacy must be respected, and a glut of unrefined, unevaluated data is of little utility. Strong interaction at the planning stage between data gatherers and information users is essential.

[201]U. S. Consumer Product Safety Commission, "NEISS: An Overview," *NEISS News 3*, #5, (April, 1975).

[202]This topic is the subject of current congressional debate, and proposals for surveillance systems are being developed by the National Bureau of Standards as authorized by the *Fire Research and Safety Act of 1968*.

[203]Matthew Meselson, in preface to *Chemical Mutagens*, edited by Alexander Hollaender (Plenum Press, New York, 1971); see also James F. Crow, "Human population monitoring," *ibid.*, Vol. 2, 591ff.

PAYING FOR IT

Because it is obvious that every aspect of making safe has its costs, and because detailed discussion is beyond our present scope, we will simply mention a few general aspects of the costs of safety.

A consideration in every public decision is how much to internalize the costs—that is, how extensively to extract the costs specifically from those who benefit. Until recently, pollution has largely been allowed to continue as an external cost; those who polluted could make their profits without paying to control the pollution, but the general public, which got little of the monetary benefit, had to pay high health and other costs. That trend is changing; polluters are increasingly being required to invest in expensive controlling equipment and personnel. But such costs as inspection and monitoring, public interest group and advocate intervention, insurance and workman's compensation, may be high and yet difficult to internalize.

With consumer products, the initial sale levies upon the buyer most of the cost of research, development, manufacture, quality control, and so on, as well as the costs of injury and ill health incurred in manufacture. Wrongly injured persons can recoup some health costs, perhaps from the manufacturer in a liability suit, or from an insuror.

These and other costs constitute the "social overhead" of a highly integrated society. The costs of maintaining a government regulatory establishment are paid for by taxes from all for the benefit of all, as are most of the costs of operating the courts that hear some several hundred thousand product liability suits and other safety cases every year.[204]

In each given case, one of the questions that must be asked is whether the distribution of costs should be decided by regulation or by redress. Should the agencies direct spending on design, development, and quality control by enforcing standards, thus using the public purse to purchase preventive action? Or should the courts distribute justice in their slow but time-honored way to influence manufacturer action indirectly? Both are flawed: the agencies are slow, inflexible, cumbersome, and vulnerable to improper influence; and the courts are slow, cumbersome, not equally available to all, and act principally after injury has already been suffered. The

---

[204]See James M. Brown, "Probing the law and beyond: A quest for public protection from hazardous product catastrophes," Staff discussion paper 402, George Washington University Program of Policy Studies in Science and Technology, National Technical Information Service, PB 192558 (1969); Guido Calabresi, *The Costs of Accidents: A Legal and Economic Analysis* (Yale University Press, New Haven, 1970); John Prather Brown, "Toward an economic theory of liability," *Journal of Legal Studies*, 323-349 (1973).

answer to the question varies with the situation.[205] Costs of research, development, testing, and licensing can be very high, as they are with pharmaceuticals; they may even be so high as to discourage introduction of new products.[206] In other instances, as the National Commission on Product Safety's *Final Report* stated,[207]

> We found that in many instances it cost little or nothing to remove or reduce the risk in certain products and that safety features may be marketed with little or no additional cost to the consumer. For example: The magnetic latch on refrigerators, to prevent entrapment, adds nothing to the consumer's cost. A double-insulated drill sells in the same price bracket as other top-line drills without double insulation. The manufacturer says the double insulation added little to his costs. TV sets whose fire records were below average sold in the same price range as those above the average. The wringer washer judged to have the safest instinctive release by Consumers Union sells at about the same price as others tested. In certain categories of consumer goods, such as electric heaters and power tools, some high-priced models have been found to be more hazardous than competing models sold at lower prices.

[205]For consumer products, two different views are presented in the National Commission on Product Safety, *Final Report* (June, 1970), and Walter Y. Oi, "The economics of product safety," *The Bell Journal of Economics and Management Science 4*, 3-28 (1973). An excellent review of cost arguments appears in James W. Singer, "Product safety efforts challenged as being too costly," *National Journal Reports*, 658-668 (May 3, 1975).

[206]President's Science Advisory Committee, *Chemicals and Health* (1973).

[207]National Commission on Product Safety, *Final Report*, 67 (1970).

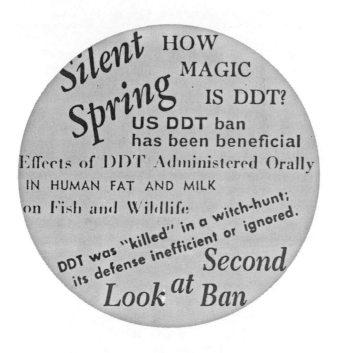

Silent Spring

HOW MAGIC IS DDT?

US DDT ban has been beneficial

Effects of DDT Administered Orally

IN HUMAN FAT AND MILK

on Fish and Wildlife

DDT was "killed" in a witch-hunt; its defense inefficient or ignored.

Second Look at Ban

6

DDT: An Archetypal Modern Problem

Throughout all four hectic decades of its history DDT has been representative of a large and proliferating class of issues that, because of their complexion as well as their contemporaneity, can appropriately be called "modern." No matter what one thinks of the particular technical and political decisions that have been made regarding it, the DDT problem richly illustrates many of the points developed in the present text.

In his 1948 acceptance of the Nobel Prize for the discovery of DDT, Paul H. Müller, of the Swiss firm J. R. Geigy, reminisced:

> When, in about 1935 . . . I began to study the field of insecticides, and in particular those insecticides of importance to agriculture, the situation looked desperate indeed. Already an immense amount of literature existed on the subject and a flood of patents had been taken out. Yet of the many patented pesticides there were practically none on the market and my own investigations showed that they were not comparable with known insecticides such as the arsenates, pyrethrum or rotenone . . . I soon realized that a contact or 'touch' insecticide would possess very much better prospects than an oral poison . . ."[208]

Müller had proceeded to test hundreds of chemicals by spraying them into large glass chambers containing houseflies or other insects and counting the kill. As the observations accumulated, he eventually noticed that a certain type of chlorinated hydrocarbon consistently seemed much more effective than other substances. Influenced by the research of other laboratories in synthetic chemistry and in mothproofing, he subjected many close relatives of the promising chemical to his tests.

The search narrowed. Less promising compounds were shelved. Finally, in 1939, a chemical whose preparation had been in the literature since 1873 (in the doctoral dissertation of an Austrian student named Othmar Zeidler) but which had been considered as of passing academic interest only and never as an insecticide, proved amazingly effective in the fly chambers: dichloro-diphenyl-trichloroethane, soon to become known around the world simply as DDT.

Müller found DDT to be extraordinarily potent: "My fly cage was so toxic after a period that even after very thorough cleaning of the cage, untreated flies, on touching the walls, fell to the floor. I could carry on my trials only after dismantling the cage, having it thoroughly cleaned and after that leaving it for about one month in the open air." The Geigy company provided samples of DDT to the Swiss Army and the Red Cross, whose field tests were extremely encouraging.[209]

For a world embroiled in its second global war, the need for a persistent general pesticide was urgent. The inevitable spread of typhus by body lice, malaria by mosquitoes, and typhoid and dysentery by flies threatened once

[208]Paul H. Müller, *Nobel Lectures: Physiology or Medicine, 1942-1962, 288* (published for the Nobel Foundation by Elsevier, New York, 1954).

[209]The Geigy involvement is described in A. Buxtorf and M. Spindler, editors, English version by G. H. de C. Ireland and R. Truan, *15 Years of Geigy Pest Control* (J. R. Geigy S.A., Basle, 1954).

again, as in every previous war, to take a greater toll of combatants and civilians alike than did bullets, bayonets, and bombs. DDT was to prove a potent weapon against the carrier insects and therefore critical for control of the diseases. It was also to prove more efficacious than the two most commonly used natural insecticides, pyrethrin (from oriental chrysanthemums) and rotenone (from various plant roots), whose supply from the Orient was cut off.

In 1942, at about the time Geigy obtained its patents, the Allies became aware of the chemical's promise. As the British entomologist V. B. Wigglesworth recollected a few years later,

> In England we read those patents and were frankly skeptical. It seemed to us that too much was claimed. The new insecticide appeared to be so exactly what we wanted that it looked too good to be true. But clearly the stuff should be tested . . . The Swiss claims were fully substantiated . . . New ways of using DDT were discovered, as it seemed, almost daily—until both British and American entomologists almost came to feel that they had discovered the stuff.[210]

Extensive tests were run on both sides of the Atlantic. DDT's insect "knock-down" performance remained impressive, and its acute toxicity was judged manageable with proper use. Production of the chemical—which had never before been an item of commerce—was ordered immediately; the United States War Production Board conferred upon DDT the same AA1 priority as penicillin. Early in 1944 Vannevar Bush, director of the United States Office of Scientific Research and Development, recommended the formation of a national DDT Committee under the supervision of the Surgeon General to coordinate research and production. The technical problems were rapidly solved, and production of DDT expanded from 1000 pounds during May 1943, to 550,000 pounds per month a year later, to almost 3,000,000 pounds per month by mid-1945.[211]

In the theaters of the war DDT was dramatically effective in preventing typhus, about which the bacteriologist and historian of medicine Hans Zinsser had lamented in 1935: "In its tragic relationship to mankind this disease is second to none—not even to plague or cholera . . ."[212] Typhus

---

[210]V. B. Wigglesworth, "DDT and the Balance of Nature," *Atlantic Monthly 176*, 107-113 (1945).

[211]U. S. Army, Medical Department, Col. John Boyd Coates, Jr., editor in chief, *Preventive Medicine in World War II*, vol. II, 257-362 (U. S. Army Medical Service, 1955).

[212]Hans Zinsser, *Rats, Lice and History*, vii, (Little, Brown and Co., Boston, 1935).

was cropping up in prison camps, in military bivouacs, in refugee camps, wherever misery harbored lice. Several public health campaigns sponsored by large American foundations used the pesticide to great advantage in aiding war-torn cities:

> Shortly after its capture by the Allied Armies in 1943, Naples was threatened by a serious epidemic of typhus. The number of cases was multiplying so rapidly that the situation was ripe for an explosive outburst of the disease. At the invitation of the United States Typhus Commission, the Rockefeller Foundation undertook the responsibility for the mass delousing of the population. Forty delousing stations were established in the city, and to these stations the people came by the thousands and tens of thousands. At each station there was a staff of men dusters to care for the boys and men, and a staff of women to care for the girls and women. DDT had by this time come into use and after careful test had superseded the other insecticides. The powder was applied directly by compressed-air guns which swoshed it up trousers and skirts, down sleeves, into collars, seams, tucks, and folds, wherever the insect or its eggs might cling. More than 1,300,000 people were treated in a single month, and the epidemic which might have taken thousands of lives collapsed with astonishing rapidity.[213]

Rushed into service by the British in the jungles of Burma, dispersed from C-47's over Saipan against an epidemic of dengue fever, sprayed on the beachhead of Morotai on D-day, DDT slashed the incidence of insect-borne diseases. Wherever the troops went, the powder was taken along: "Soldiers and sailors by the million carried small cans of DDT powder to protect themselves against bedbugs, lice, and mosquitoes. They came to love the stuff, especially in the tropics. Millions of DDT aerosol bombs were used to spray the interiors of tents, barracks, and mess halls. Through European refugee camps, along the Burma Road, across jungle battlefields of Southeast Asia, on Saipan and dozens of South Sea isles infested by stinging, biting insects, DDT spread its beneficent mist."[214]

At the end of the hostilities these duly impressed troops returned home and avidly began to adopt the versatile dust for general use around their homes and farms.

The wartime and postwar accomplishments of DDT against both disease-carrying and crop-destroying insects are universally acknowledged. The chemical was efficacious, certainly, and it seemed to be relatively safe.

---

[213]Raymond Fosdick, *The Story of the Rockefeller Foundation*, 50 (Harper & Brothers, New York, 1952).

[214]Kenneth S. Davis, "The Deadly Dust: The unhappy history of DDT," *American Heritage* 22, no. 2, 45 (1971).

Any timid warnings of ill side effects were likely to be dismissed, or even ridiculed, as in the following *Saturday Evening Post* article by Brigadier General James Stevens Simmons, the Chief of the U. S. Army's Preventive Medicine Service:

> Armed with DDT, the Army has conquered the fear of typhus. For the first time in history, this ruthless companion of disaster, famine and poverty has lost all right to its murderous title of champion of the ancient plagues of war . . . Meanwhile these reports of the amazing uses of DDT are passed over for yarns telling of its destructiveness which sound like newly created versions of the Arabian Nights. These incredible rumors picture DDT as a substance which may bring complete ruin to both the animal and the vegetable kingdoms. For example, a serious scientific report that DDT has killed millions of mosquito larvae in Gatun Lake may be overshadowed by a fantastic story claiming that particles of the chemicals, transported by the winds, have annihilated all the blue butterflies in the Isthmus of Darien.[215]

Extensive tests of acute toxicity had been carried out during the war by the chemical manufacturers and by the Department of Agriculture, and they continued after the war. In one series of tests, for example, the Agricultural Research Administration studied the effects of feeding large doses of DDT to cows, horses, and sheep (and unintentionally to an ill-fated English sparrow that wandered into the barn, ate some DDT-treated grain, and died). Added daily to feed at levels of 100 milligrams of DDT powder per kilogram animal body weight (or about 1½ ounces of DDT daily for a 1000-pound cow), the pesticide was shown to induce loss of appetite and scattered hemorrhaging. Several cows "developed rather marked tremors, especially in the hind legs and necks, and showed a tendency to lift their hind feet as if the leg muscles or feet were sore. . . . They also became much more excitable than usual, and their eyes assumed a wild or alarmed stare, especially when there was any unusual noise or activity in the barn." It was important to determine whether DDT was being passed from the cows' digestive tracts into their bloodstreams or whether it was simply being excreted, but reliable methods for measuring DDT chemically had not yet been developed. The best that could be done was to place blood samples from the cows in screen cages containing houseflies and allow the flies to feed on the blood. In 24 hours, blood from a cow fed DDT killed 50 percent of the flies in its cage, whereas in a control cage containing blood from a

---

[215]Brig. Gen. James Stevens Simmons, "How Magic is DDT?" *Saturday Evening Post 217*, 18 (January 6, 1945).

cow not fed DDT, less than 2 percent of the flies died, thus allowing the conclusion that DDT was indeed passing into the bloodstream.[216]

Nevertheless, since the amounts of DDT used in the tests were enormous compared to the amounts to which livestock and humans would normally be exposed, there seemed to be little cause for alarm and DDT was generally regarded to be safe for humans.

There were indeed some public warnings, but because of the tenuous nature of the evidence they were mostly quite mild. As early as March 1945, the Department of Agriculture cautioned that "Too little is yet known about the harm that DDT may do to beneficial insects, plants, soil, livestock, wildlife, or to consumers of fruit and vegetables containing DDT residues."[217] In a postwar transition period bulletin of "Suggestions regarding the use of DDT by civilians" the Department of Agriculture cautiously warned that

> DDT is harmful to honeybees and other beneficial insects, as are a number of other insecticides. Used indiscriminatingly, DDT may interfere with adequate pollination of important food or seed crop plants and destroy beneficial insect parasites and predators that ordinarily keep certain injurious pests under control. DDT is highly toxic to fish and certain other cold-blooded animals, but is much less poisonous to warm-blooded animals. Under certain conditions its use experimentally has resulted in some killing of insect-feeding birds . . .[218]

And in reporting their extensive field studies of the effects of DDT on fish and wildlife, Department of the Interior scientists warned that it "like every other effective insecticide or rodenticide, is really a two-edged sword."[219] But these well-meant statements caused little alarm and were taken mostly as routine disclaimers of the sort that usually accompany the introduction of any promising new technology. The military emergency had been met; the diseases of war had been controlled. For a world newly aware of the interdependence of its parts, DDT was especially important for protecting the international food supply from the ravages of insects. DDT improved

---

[216]L. W. Orr and L. O. Mott, *Journal of Economic Entomology 38,* 428-432 (1945).

[217]U. S. Department of Agriculture, "Some facts about DDT insecticides to date—Some of the results of two years' testing," *U.S.D.A. bulletin 503-45* (March 20, 1945).

[218]U. S. Department of Agriculture, "Suggestions regarding the use of DDT by civilians," *U.S.D.A. bulletin 2574-45-1* (August 22, 1945).

[219]C. Cotton, "DDT and its effects on fish and wildlife," *Journal of Economic Entomology 39,* 44-52 (1946).

crop yields and kept household pests in check; it was useful not only against mosquitoes, flies, and lice, but also against a whole assortment of beetles, thrips, cankerworms, boll weevils and bollworms, moths, and caterpillars. It was effective, easy to apply, and cheap.

Initially, the overall public assessment of DDT was that its benefits far exceeded its detriments. About the only people thought to be at risk were spraymen and a few manufacturing workers. The hazards were seen as short-term and caused largely by misuse, and they could be controlled: warning labels were put on containers; farm workers were instructed on when and how to spray; methods were advised for washing fruit; the Food and Drug Administration set limits for permissible concentrations in food; and analytical methods were developed for monitoring residues in food and in the environment. The many animal experiments had been reassuring about all but massive doses of the chemical; occupational and accidental exposures had not had alarming consequences; and deliberate human feeding experiments had revealed no confirmable ill effects. Little serious harm came from the occasional inefficacy incurred as a few insects became resistant to DDT, since those pests could be controlled by other measures.

In order to manage the problems associated with the growing use of DDT and the burgeoning variety of other new pest control agents coming onto the market, such as aldin and dieldrin, hexachlorobenzene, and the organophosphates, the Congress in 1947 passed the Federal Insecticide, Fungicide, and Rodenticide Act. This Act tightened existing regulations somewhat, providing among several new requirements that these chemicals be registered with the Department of Agriculture prior to being marketed. As much as for any other purpose, the Act was intended to protect "progressive" farmers from misleading claims and unsafe and inefficacious products as they modernized their farming.

As the use of DDT expanded, after animal studies had indicated the range of effect, several series of human experiments were carried out. A study often referred to is that conducted by Wayland J. Hayes and his colleagues at the Public Health Service's Communicable Disease Center in Atlanta. They summarized their report as follows: "With full knowledge of the plan of the study and with complete freedom to withdraw at any time, 51 men (inmates of a federal correctional institution) volunteered to take daily, oral doses of DDT for different intervals. One-third of the men received no DDT except that in the ordinary diet; one-third received 3.5 mg. per man per day; and one-third received 35 mg. per man per day, which is about 200 times the daily rate at which an average man received DDT from his diet. During the entire study, no volunteer complained of any symptom or showed, by the tests used, any sign of illness that did not have an easily recognized cause clearly unrelated to exposure to DDT."[220]

Although alternative chemicals were becoming available, largely because of its physical persistence and low cost DDT continued to be sprayed by the millions of pounds onto the land through the 1950s and into the 1960s. Then the situation began to change.

Joltingly, and for perhaps the first time, man was to learn from DDT that he had contaminated to a demonstrable degree the entire land, air, and water masses of his globe, his food supply, and indeed his own flesh, with a chemical of his own manufacture. Although this dubious distinction may instead belong to the radioactive fallout from the early atmospheric nuclear weapons detonations, or even earlier, to lead, DDT was probably the first case in which the general public became aware and became involved.

For most people the news was delivered in 1962 by Rachel Carson's *Silent Spring*.[221] To a public accustomed to taking DDT for granted as a great benefit, the contrary view came as an upsetting surprise. *Silent Spring* first appeared in abridged form as a three-part series in *The New Yorker*; the book itself became an immediate best-seller and a selection of the Book-of-the-Month Club. Its paperbound edition went on to catch the attention of countless conservation enthusiasts, college students, and housewives.[222]

Silent Spring was extremely well written. Carson, a biologist with a master's degree, had pursued her research carefully, as she had earlier with her books *Under the Sea Wind* and *The Sea Around Us*. Every point was documented. Developing its exposition from images of a sterilized earth, the book conveyed an emotional effect that other writings of its kind had not. Although its merits were hotly debated, and although it certainly had shortcomings, the book did provide an alarming inventory of the distribution of this persistent, traveling chemical. DDT was everywhere on the surface of the earth. DDT was in every body of air and water. DDT was in the bodies of virtually all living creatures. DDT was in man's own flesh.

---

[220]W. J. Hayes, Jr., W. F. Durham, and C. Cueto, Jr., "The effects of known repeated oral doses of chlorophenothane (DDT) in man," *Journal of the American Medical Association 162*, 890-897 (1956); Wayland J. Hayes, Jr., William E. Hale, and Carl I. Pirkle, "Evidence of safety of long-term, high oral doses of DDT for man," *Archives of Environmental Health 22*, 119-135 (1971); a review of the problems encountered in such testing appears in Wayland J. Hayes, Jr., "Tests in man," in *Modern Trends in Toxicology*, 198-230 (E. Boyland, editor, Appleton-Century-Crofts, New York, 1968).

[221]Rachel Carson, *Silent Spring* (Houghton Mifflin, Boston, 1962).

[222]For an account of the publishing history of the book, see Frank Graham, Jr., *Since Silent Spring* (Houghton Mifflin, Boston, 1970).

Carson pointed out that the hundreds of millions of pounds of DDT that had been released around the world in the years since its discovery had been redistributed so broadly from their immediate point of application that they had infiltrated the tissues of every human on earth. In her words:

> Storage in human beings has been well investigated, and we know that the average person is storing potentially harmful amounts. According to various studies, individuals with no known exposure (except the inevitable dietary one) store an average of 5.3 parts per million to 7.4 parts per million; agricultural workers 17.1 parts per million; and workers in insecticide plants as high as 648 parts per million! So the range of proven storage is quite wide and, what is even more to the point, the minimum figures are above the level at which damage to the liver and other organs or tissues may begin.

(Notice that the progress in analytical chemistry since the days of the crude housefly assays allowed her to speak of measurements of parts per million.) And furthermore, since DDT is more soluble in fatty tissues than in non-fatty ones, it becomes greatly concentrated:

> The fatty storage depots act as biological magnifiers, so that an intake of as little as 1/10 of 1 part per million in the diet results in storage of about 10 to 15 parts per million, an increase of one-hundredfold or more.

And since DDT may take years to deteriorate, it can be dispersed by the winds and the waters, and in a special way by living organisms:

> One of the most sinister features of DDT and related chemicals is the way they are passed on from one organism to another through all the links of the food chains. For example, fields of alfalfa are dusted with DDT; meal is later prepared from the alfalfa and fed to hens; the hens lay eggs which contain DDT. Or the hay, containing residues of 7 to 8 parts per million, may be fed to cows. The DDT will turn up in the milk in the amount of about 3 parts per million, but in butter made from this milk the concentration may run to 65 parts per million. Through such a process of transfer, what started out as a very small amount of DDT may end as a heavy concentration . . . There has been no such parallel situation in medical history. No one yet knows what the ultimate consequences may be.

Much of *Silent Spring* dealt with the poisonous effects of the chemicals on wildlife and the circumstances which had suggested the book's mournful title.

> Large residues of DDT and other [polychlorinated] hydrocarbons have been found whenever looked for in the eggs of birds subjected to these chemicals,

163

either experimentally or in the wild. And the concentrations have been heavy. Pheasant eggs in a California experiment contained up to 349 parts per million of DDT. In Michigan, eggs taken from the oviducts of robins dead of DDT poisoning showed concentrations up to 200 parts per million. Other eggs were taken from nests unattended as parent robins were stricken with poison; these too contained DDT.

This grim vision of a world sterilized by man's unknowing hand, this tale of dying robins and sickly salmon, caught the attention of a sympathetic public. The book was boosted by heavy press coverage; in the first ten months after its publication, the *New York Times* carried stories about it on twenty-three separate occasions. It was a case in which the mass media played a key role in amplifying a controversy triggered by a crusader:

> The coverage by the *New York Times* as the issues unfolded served many purposes. The public was educated on the benefits and detriments of pesticides. The institutions behind the controversy were illuminated and their interests explained. Those who faithfully followed each step saw the tempo increase and a climax approaching. Finally, and most importantly, by generally supporting Rachel Carson's arguments, the *Times* added its prestige and influence to the call for reform and new legislation.[223]

This is not to say that the book was without fault. Many detractors— by no means all of them representing agricultural or chemical manufacturing interests—took Carson to task for presenting only the bad effects of DDT and neglecting its benefits in controlling crop pests and insect-borne infectious diseases. Reviewing the book in the magazine *Science,* I. L. Baldwin, professor of agricultural bacteriology at the University of Wisconsin and chairman of the Committee on Pest Control and Wildlife Relationships of the National Research Council, said that

> *Silent Spring* is superbly written and beautifully illustrated with line drawings. The author has made an exhaustive study of the facts bearing on the problem. It is not, however, a judicial review or a balancing of the gains and losses; rather, it is the prosecuting attorney's impassioned plea for action against the use of these new materials which have received such widespread acceptance, acceptance accorded because of the obvious benefits that their use has conferred.[224]

---

[223]Dennis W. Brezina, "The role of crusader-triggered controversy in technology assessment: An analysis of the mass media response to *Silent Spring* and *Unsafe At Any Speed,*" George Washington University Program in Policy Studies in Science and Technology, staff discussion paper 203, 1968, available as publication PB 182875 of the National Technical Information Service.

[224]I. L. Baldwin, *Science 137,* 1042 (1962).

Cornell University biologist LaMont C. Cole also gave it a mixed review, commenting in *Scientific American*: "As an ecologist I am glad this provocative book has been written. That is not to say I consider it a fair and impartial appraisal of all the evidence. On the contrary, it is a highly partisan selection of examples and interpretations that support the author's theses."[225]

Prompted at least indirectly by the controversy over *Silent Spring*, a panel of President Kennedy's Science Advisory Committee (PSAC) conducted a careful study of the use of pesticides. Citing the value of heightened public awareness of these difficult issues, the committee report acknowledged that "Public literature and the experiences of Panel members indicate that, until the publication of 'Silent Spring' by Rachel Carson, people were generally unaware of the toxicity of pesticides."[226] This PSAC report, released in 1963, summarized a large body of published research in saying:

> Today, pesticides are detectable in many food items, in some clothing, in man and animals, and in various parts of our natural surroundings. Carried from one locality to another by air currents, water runoff, or living organisms (either directly or indirectly through extended food chains), pesticides have traveled great distances and some of them have persisted for long periods of time. Although they remain in small quantities, their variety, toxicity, and persistence are affecting biological systems in nature and may eventually affect human health. The benefits of these substances are apparent. We are now beginning to evaluate some of their less obvious effects and potential risks.[227]

The Committee called for rapid, intensive study of the toxicity of the pesticides; for review and, if necessary, reorganization of federal programs of research, regulation, and monitoring; and for a program of public education. Its controversial recommendation, that "elimination of the use of *persistent* toxic pesticides should be the goal," (emphasis added) set the tenor for much subsequent federal activity.

About the time the PSAC report was issued, an extensive series of hearings was conducted by a Senate Government Operations subcommittee chaired by Abraham Ribicoff. These hearings provided a valuable platform for many special interest groups. Particularly important testimony came from the Secretary of the Interior, Stewart L. Udall. Miss Carson "has

---

[225]LaMont C. Cole, *Scientific American 207*, #6, 173 (December, 1962).

[226]PSAC, *Use of Pesticides*, 23 (1963).

[227]PSAC, *ibid.*, 4 (1963).

awakened the Nation," Udall stated, "and has reminded us with compelling urgency that man is part of the balance of nature, man is part of the natural chain of life, and no matter how much we alter the balance, we still are a part of it." "Although her critics have protested the inadequacy of certain data cited in her book," the Secretary asserted, "they have not, to my knowledge, challenged the fact that she raises genuine issues." He went on to catalogue the Interior Department's discoveries of DDT and its chemical relatives at up to 200 parts per million in tuna and in halibut; in 1753 specimens of birds and mammals collected near Washington, D. C.; in oysters; and on and on.[228]

Silent Spring did not establish to the satisfaction of many readers the relation between dose and effect for DDT. Nor did it present a balanced view of the overall consequences of use of the pesticide. But most people felt that it had indeed raised important issues. It had inventoried the distribution of DDT and some of the conditions under which living things were being exposed to the chemical, and it had called attention to possible adverse effects of that exposure. This one rather quiet biologist, researching and writing carefully, finding powerful amplification in the media, and, perhaps, being in the right place at the right time, had touched off a debate of a magnitude that none of the other concerned postwar scientists had been able to accomplish.

How had the situation changed since, say, 1950? The problem was no longer one of acute exposure, but rather one of chronic, low-level exposure. Technological advances had made alternative methods of pest control cheaper and more effective. New analytical techniques were raising new questions. And whereas at first the problem had been mostly one of free choice for farmers and a few public health experts, it was gaining urgency as a problem affecting everyone on the earth. The environmental battle was clashingly joined, and the word "ecology" was newly added to the everyday vocabulary. The questions of such human health effects as carcinogenesis, although less compelling presented, were nevertheless raised.

The years following were a time of reassessment. How correct had Rachel Carson been? Even if some portions of her evidence were to prove insubstantial, her admonition that it was time to take stock seemed entirely valid. Various departments of the federal bureaucracy conducted reviews appropriate to their jurisdiction: Agriculture developed advice on farm use,

---

[228]U. S. Senate Subcommittee on Reorganization and International Organizations of the Committee on Government Operations, *Hearings on Interagency Coordination in Environmental Hazards (Pesticides)*, 1963-1964.

Interior reviewed forestry and other applications, the Food and Drug Administration revised some food tolerances—a survey of the bureaus' responses to *Silent Spring* and to the 1963 PSAC recommendations would make a fascinating review in itself.

Two particularly important studies were undertaken by the Department of Health, Education, and Welfare. Through its National Cancer Institute, HEW contracted with the private Bionetics Research Laboratories to study the carcinogenicity of some common pesticides; DDT would eventually prove carcinogenic to some animals under certain test conditions. And HEW Secretary Robert Finch convened a Commission on Pesticides and Their Relationship to Environmental Health, chaired by Emil Mrak of the University of California at Davis. The Commission's report, issued in late 1969, was a remarkably balanced and comprehensive document. After reviewing all the available evidence regarding both ecological and medical effects, it made the strong recommendation that the nation "eliminate within two years all uses of DDT . . . in the United States excepting those uses essential to the preservation of human health or welfare and approved unanimously by the Secretaries of the Department of Health, Education, and Welfare, Agriculture, and Interior." Running through all 577 pages of the report, however, were *caveats* and reminders that the facts were exceedingly difficult to pin down. The chapter prepared by the Panel on Carcinogenicity is reminiscent of our second chapter:

> The evidence for the carcinogenicity of DDT in experimental animals is impressive and the Panel takes no exception to the conclusions as to DDT recorded in the [Bionetics] report of the National Cancer Institute study. *This study has demonstrated that DDT increased the incidence of cancer in mice under the experimental conditions employed. However, this does not prove carcinogenicity for human beings at the very much lower levels to which they are actually exposed.*
>
> Since tests with groups of laboratory animals comparable in size to large populations of humans are impractical, and because wide species differences exist, high levels of exposure are used. Whether or not this device is adequate for extrapolation from experimental results to the human situation remains very uncertain, for research on induced cancer is replete with examples of differences in responses of different species to various carcinogens. Furthermore the metabolism of many chemicals varies with dosage level.
>
> Evaluation of human experience with DDT has revealed little if any evidence of long-term adverse health effects from its use. On the other hand, the observations of human experience have not been sufficient to eliminate the possibility that continued chronic exposure may slowly induce a low level of cancer in man . . .

167

Accordingly, with the evidence now in, DDT can be regarded neither as a proven danger as a carcinogen for man nor as an assuredly safe pesticide; suspicion has been aroused and it should be confirmed or dispelled.

In the resolution of this issue, mere repetition of the tests conducted at Bionetics Research Laboratories would be of only limited value. Of greater importance will be:

1. Studies conducted on several animal species,

2. A much more critical study of human experience,

3. Development of knowledge relative to comparative metabolism and factors controlling dose-response relationships which may reinforce and improve ability to extrapolate from the findings of animal studies to man,

4. Studies on very large groups of animals, at a range of dose levels including those comparable to human exposure,

5. Evaluation of interaction of or potentiation of DDT with or by other materials, and

6. Studies of the tumorigenicity of DDT administered to several successive generations of one or more animal species.[229]

During the 1960s, much research attention was focused on DDT: Where had it traveled? How fast did it decay? Did it really cause thinning of eggshells and other ecological damage? Could it really cause cancer? At the same time, alternative, less persistent pesticides continued to be developed, as were strategies for nonchemical insect control. State and local governments held public hearings and began to take regulatory actions. However, very little federal action was taken.

The year 1969 brought a critical development. The Environmental Defense Fund (EDF), a public interest group which had gained valuable experience in court battles over DDT in New York, Michigan, and Wisconsin, losing some of its court fights but gaining considerable public sympathy for its cause, mounted a direct attack on the federal government's stance on DDT. The EDF and its allies petitioned the Department of Agriculture to order the suspension of the use of DDT. Complicated legal maneuvering by both sides eventually culminated in a U. S. Court of Appeals directive for the Department of Agriculture to ban DDT. At just that crucial moment all responsibility for the regulation of pesticides was reassigned to the newly formed Environmental Protection Agency (EPA), established by Executive initiative in 1970 and headed by William D. Ruckelshaus.

---

[229]Department of Health, Education, and Welfare, *Report of the Secretary's Commission on Pesticides and Their Relationship to Environmental Health*, 471 (1969).

The Court of Appeals ordered the EPA to take action against DDT. Over the next two years the shudders of the collision reverberated: cancellation (temporary banning) of DDT by the EPA; appeal of the cancellation by the manufacturers; review by advisory committees; a court order to EPA to consider suspension (permanent banning) of DDT; hearings requested by the manufacturers; the hearing examiner's recommending that the cancellation be lifted—and finally, Ruckelshaus ordering, with minor exceptions, full suspension of crop and non-health use of DDT, effective by the end of 1972.[230]

In a large part of the world, especially in the developing tropical nations, the continuing low-budget battles against famine and disease have led to entirely different judgments about DDT. This inexpensive pesticide is finding increasing use against the insect carriers of onchocerciasis, trypanosomiasis, filariasis, and other dread tropical diseases rarely encountered in the United States. The World Health Organization continues to support the use of DDT; as one of its expert committees reiterated in 1973,

> The predominant use of DDT in public health is still for malaria eradication. More than 1000 million people are now living in areas that have been freed from the endemic form of the disease. However, it is becoming increasingly clear that to maintain this achievement and to permit the extension of protection to the many millions of persons still exposed to infection will require the continued availability of DDT. The withdrawal of this compound from public health use at this time could give rise to immense problems and expose large populations to outbreaks of endemic and epidemic malaria.[231]

In the United States the use of DDT is severely restricted by government regulations. The first major exception to the EPA ban was made in March 1974, to allow DDT to be used against the tussock moth. The furry larvae of this moth were eating their way through the beautiful and commercially important fir timber of the northwestern states—stripping the

---

[230]U. S. Environmental Protection Agency, "Consolidated DDT hearings, opinion and order of the Administrator," 37 Federal Register, 13369-13375 (July 7, 1972); Frank Graham, Jr., Since Silent Spring (Houghton Mifflin Company, Boston, 1970); Luther J. Carter, "Environmental law: Maturing field for lawyers and scientists," Science 179, 1205-1209, 1310-1312, 1350 (1973); John E. Blodgett, "Pesticides: Regulation of an evolving technology," in Samuel S. Epstein and Richard D. Grundy, editors, Consumer Health and Product Hazards, vol. 2, 197-288 (MIT Press, Cambridge, 1974); Joel Primack and Frank von Hippel, "The battle over persistent pesticides: From Rachel Carson to the Environmental Defense Fund," in their Advice and Dissent: Scientists in the Political Arena (Basic Books, New York, 1974); Rita Gray Beatty, The DDT Myth. Triumph of the Amateurs (The John Day Company, New York, 1973).

[231]World Health Organization Expert Committee on Insecticides, "Safe use of pesticides," WHO Technical Report No. 513 (Geneva, 1973).

foliage from more than 589,000 acres of timber in Washington and Oregon in 1973, often with lethal effect—and a hoped-for epidemic of the moth's natural nemesis, the tussock moth virus, which usually keeps the moths in check, failed to arise. Chemicals other than DDT were reported to be ineffective. Methods for growing the virus in the laboratory were not yet promising.[232] Timber producers, farmers, and the Forest Service petitioned for use of DDT. In a difficult decision, EPA administrator Russell Train granted emergency use of DDT if, in the opinion of the Forest Service, "the use of DDT cannot be avoided." Interviewed by *Science* magazine, Train described the decision:

> *Q. Some environmentalists, although they may give you high marks generally, have felt that in certain of your decisions you have yielded to political pressures that should have been resisted. Your recent decision to allow the Forest Service to use DDT for control of the tussock moth in the Northwest this year has been cited as a case in point. What is your reply to such criticism?*
>
> Train: I guess the decision in the tussock moth case was one of the toughest I've had to make, maybe the toughest. Certainly it was an unhappy decision—for anybody who has been in the environmental business as long as I have—to approve use of DDT, even though the approval carried strict conditions. I emphasized at the time the decision was made that it should in no way be taken as signaling any pullback from the agency's basic position that DDT is an environmental threat. The issue here is, first, whether there was an emergency, and, second, whether there was any alternative . . . Now, there is no question but what the public in the Northwest perceives this situation as an emergency. It is true everywhere you go out there . . . I don't think it was a matter, as some would say, of giving way to pressure. Public perceptions of problems such as this are very important in carrying out a regulatory program, particularly when you have mixed scientific evidence.
>
> *Q: You think there was no clear-cut preponderance of scientific opinion on one side or the other?*
>
> Train: I would say not.[233]

The general dispute will continue. From time to time various American scientists urge exoneration of DDT. Others argue strongly for elimination not only of DDT but of all its chemical relatives as well. Production of DDT in the United States has fallen off to very low levels; at present only one American company is manufacturing the chemical, most of it for export.

---

[232]U. S. Environmental Protection Agency, "The Douglas fir tussock moth in the Pacific Northwest," a seminar in Seattle sponsored by the Environmental Protection Agency (November 16, 1973).

[233]"Russell E. Train: Speaking out at EPA," *Science 184*, 139-140 (April 12, 1974).

Recently, the shortage of DDT was lamented by the World Health Organization's Southeast Asia Regional Committee in a resolution warning of a "recrudescence of malaria in epidemic form . . . particularly in Bangladesh, Burma, India, Indonesia, Maldives, Nepal, Sri Lanka, and Thailand . . . primarily due to the inadequate and delayed supply of insecticides, particularly DDT, which, in turn, is due to inadequate manufacturing capacity within the region and also to the prohibitive cost and limited supply from developed counties."[234]

For many uses of DDT in protecting both crops and human health, chemical alternatives are now readily available, at least to developed nations that can pay the higher prices. Many of these other pesticides are at least as efficacious as DDT and are more species-specific. But many are of greater acute toxicity, posing a danger to manufacturers and spraymen. And we may later find that they, too, bring unacceptably high chronic risks; with some of them, we have not yet had enough experience to know. Biological agents such as sterilized predator beetles (which attack their natural insect prey voraciously during their one-generation existence) and species-specific viruses (which decimate particular insect populations by their infection but do not harm other species) are being developed, but progress has been disappointingly slow. The very success of DDT, along with its low price and the subtlety of its adverse effects, has doubtless in some ways inhibited the development of alternatives.

Even now, more than thirty-five years after the discovery of DDT, we still don't understand its risks satisfactorily. More than thirty years after the first ecological warnings, we still don't really understand how it affects the environment, how fast it decays, whether it causes eggshell thinning, or whether it affects the plants and animals of the oceans; most observers, however, are convinced that it does have important environmental effects. More than twenty-seven years after the first suspicion over its carcinogenicity, scientists in many nations are still trying to determine whether low exposures to it can cause human cancer. Experiments have recently shown that under certain conditions DDT does induce liver tumors in mice.[235]

DDT has been extensively tested on humans. That studies on other species would never be so convincing has been emphasized by a panel advising the Secretary of Health, Education, and Welfare:

[234]World Health Organization, "Anti-malaria programme," resolution SEA/RC27/Min. 5 (September 6, 1974).

[235]L. Tomatis, V. Turusov, N. Day, and R. T. Charles, "The effect of long-term exposure to DDT on CF-1 mice," *International Journal of Cancer 10*, 489-506 (1972); L. Tomatis, V. Turusov, R. T. Charles, M. Boiocchi, and E. Gati, "Liver tumours in CF-1 mice exposed for limited periods to technical DDT," *Zeitschrift für Krebsforschung 82*, 25-35 (1974).

Controlled exposure of human volunteers to pesticides under close medical supervision constitutes the most reliable approach to the unequivocal evaluation of long-term effects of low levels of pesticide exposure. The difficulties involved in maintaining such studies have inevitably resulted in very small groups of subjects being exposed for any appreciable length of time. The longest studies on record have lasted less than four years and the results can only reflect the period of study. Consequently, the findings, especially when they are negative, are open to question when taken by themselves. It appears, however, that present levels of exposure to DDT among the general population have not produced any observable adverse effect in controlled studies on volunteers.[236]

Nor have massive occupational exposures, or accidental ingestions, even by children, been known to cause a single death anywhere in the world in the thirty-five years of DDT's history. Although this is encouraging, it does *not* rule out the possibility that some chronic human illnesses are caused, or aggravated, by the pesticide. Intensive scientific investigation continues: a check of the indexes to the world's medical and chemical literature for 1972 shows 157 citations to DDT by *Index Medicus* and 670 by *Chemical Abstracts*.

The thirty-five years' seesawing over DDT neatly demonstrates how decisions on safety are determined both by estimations of risk and by judgments of their acceptability. It demonstrates how relative the resulting decisions are, varying over time and situation. It illustrates how even problems, like our present ecological ones, that appear major when viewed with the "insight of hindsight" may in their earlier stages simply lie dormant—because they are the business of nobody in particular. The *Silent Spring* episode illustrates the influence a crusader can have; and it shows how such a person as Rachel Carson, who begins a study as an assessor, can become an advocate of a particular course, while advocates, such as some of the officials in the Agriculture and Interior departments who had championed DDT, are caused to step back and reassess.

Notice the difference *kinds* of decisions that have guided DDT's history. The earliest, wartime development decisions had mostly to do with efficacy, benefit, cost, and technical feasibility. Practical alternatives were not available. The risks, measured under emergency conditions, seemed acceptable, so safety was not a pivotal consideration. In the years after the war, when "progress" was the byword in farming and forestry as well as in chemistry, the criteria of efficacy and benefit were dominant. The search for more pest-specific, non-resistance-inducing alternatives was carried forward; but

---

[236]Department of Health, Education, and Welfare, *Report of the Secretary's Commission on Pesticides and Their Relationship to Environmental Health*, 34 (1969).

in the meantime, DDT became not only an agent for domestic use, but also, in both disease eradication and crop protection, an agent of international good will. Little appeared on the debit side of the ledger, until *Silent Spring*.

Then, of course, safety considerations became important: was the risk acceptable? Cost was important but not critical, and other beneficial alternatives were becoming available. With the realization that exposure to the pesticide had become involuntary and inescapable for every living being, questions arose about the social distribution of hazards and benefits. In the United States, detriment was weighed against benefit in many different forums. But some of the most important decisions had more to do with respect for uncertainty than with *known* characteristics. During the 1960s, apprehension about the consequences of spreading more of the stuff, irretrievably, through the global environment was heightened by the change in social values that accompanied the awakening of environmental consciousness. Alternatives to DDT seemed able to take care of the needs of most Western nations. Tough bans on DDT were widely endorsed.

Currently, we may be entering a new phase. Some of the earlier risk estimates are being challenged as being too pessimistic. Spiraling food and fiber costs are prompting reassessment, as are the famines and resurgences of malaria and other DDT-controllable diseases in several parts of the world. Humanitarian concern may very well now dictate a redistribution of costs, hazards, and benefits: increased manufacture of DDT, one of the cheapest pesticides known, in the developed nations; increased application in areas of suffering; acceptance of the still poorly understood hazard that would eventually be brought back to this end of the global food chain; investment in public health monitoring measures as a precaution at home. It remains to be seen whether alternative pest-control techniques will be developed before the above actions are deemed necessary, or whether perhaps the natural hazards of drought and disease will diminish.[237]

In any event, the saga of DDT—from the first few crystals of Paul Müller's, to the more than 4,400,000,000 pounds that have been spread around the world since then, to whatever happens in the coming years—will continue to be richly illustrative of the difficulties of resolving policy dilemmas whose solutions, it sometimes seems, are all equally unsatisfactory.

[237]U. S. Environmental Protection Agency, *DDT: A Review of Scientific and Economic Aspects of the Decision to Ban Its Use as a Pesticide*, EPA-540/1-75-022 (July, 1975).

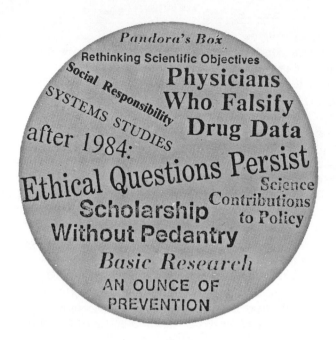

7

An Afterword

The effective afterword for this book will be the discussions that ensue in response to it.

Reaching for a diverse readership, we have essayed broadly and in a vernacular language; these explorations need to be continued with the precise techniques and specialized languages of the several intellectual disciplines. We have outlined some general schemes; they need to be tailored to particular situations. We have not dealt extensively with the questions of institutional organization, personal roles, or the just distribution of powers and burdens; those need to be addressed further, in the contexts of social legitimacy and accountability. We have resisted the temptation to confront the distracting but obviously important issues of carelessness, blindness, selfishness, and outright venality; as always, those offenses deserve to be smoked out and attacked with outraged vigor.

Our society will be at least inefficient, and at worst irresponsible, if it neglects its conceptual armament. The only hope for coping with the onrushing future is to devise defenses that are versatile: to pursue generic research and standards applicable to entire classes of products and environments; to establish scientifico-legal principles adaptable to a variety of decisional situations, obviating the need to re-erect the same evidential bridges in every new skirmish; and to employ safeguarding tactics linked explicitly to major social strategies.

There is a need to review the embodiment of the notion of acceptability in such approaches as referenda, adversary hearings, and the Delaney principle. This will no doubt raise many questions of the form, *Who should decide on acceptability of what risks for whom, and in what terms, and why?* The concept of acceptability needs to be given its proper place among considerations of cost, efficacy, and the other components of social decisions so that, for instance, it becomes commonly understood how a thing can be unsafe but perhaps unavoidable for the time being, or how a thing can be quite safe but nevertheless undesirable on other grounds.

Pervading all of these considerations is the crucial matter of the attitudes the segments of society hold toward each other. We must hope that the society at large will come to appreciate the capabilities and inherent limitations of science and technology; and we must hope that those in the technical world will come to appreciate the nonrational nature and great subtlety of social decisions.

The risks are changing. Menaces are upon us. Time is short. Decisions have to be made. . .

May discussion of these troublesome issues be temperate, imaginative, and effective.

Appendix:
Sources of Documents

National Academy of Sciences,
 National Academy of Engineering,
 National Research Council,
 Institute of Medicine
Printing and Publishing Office
2101 Constitution Avenue NW
Washington, D.C. 20418

National Technical Information Service
5285 Port Royal Road
Springfield, Virginia 22161

National Safety Council
425 North Michigan Avenue
Chicago, Illinois 60611

U.S. Product Safety Commission
Washington, D.C. 20207

U.S. Department of Health, Education,
 and Welfare
Washington, D.C. 20201

U.S. Environmental Protection Agency
401 M Street SW
Washington, D.C. 20460

U.S. Food and Drug Administration
5600 Fishers Lane
Rockville, Maryland 20852

U.S. Government Printing Office
Superintendent of Documents
Washington, D.C. 20402

U.S. National Institutes of Health
9000 Rockville Pike
Bethesda, Maryland 20014

U.S. National Institute for Occupational
 Safety and Health
5600 Fishers Lane
Rockville, Maryland 20852

U.S. Occupational Safety and Health
 Administration
Third Street and Constitution Ave. NW
Washington, D.C. 20210

Index

About the Author

William W. Lowrance is a scientist and critic who views the sciences as being among the great humanities and who approaches the issues of science in contemporary affairs with the spirit of the "natural philosophers."

He grew up in North Carolina, graduating with honors from high school in Asheville and from the University of North Carolina in Chapel Hill. After receiving his Ph.D. in organic chemistry and biochemistry in 1970 from The Rockefeller University in New York, he has pursued research in industrial chemistry, in public education, and in science and technology policy.

Of Acceptable Risk, his first book, was written while he was a Resident Fellow of the National Academy of Sciences in Washington, D.C., from 1973 to 1975; this work was supported by the Alfred P. Sloan Foundation and the National Science Foundation.

Now a Research Fellow with Harvard University's Program for Science and International Affairs, Dr. Lowrance is continuing his studies of social risk. His research interests also include the implications of worldwide nuclear power development for the proliferation of nuclear weapons, the science and technology policy problems of the United States, the ethical responsibilities of scientists, physicians, engineers and other technical specialists, and the relationships between science and art.